Viral Outbreaks - Global Impact and Newer Horizons

Edited by Shailendra K. Saxena

Published in London, United Kingdom

Viral Outbreaks - Global Impact and Newer Horizons
http://dx.doi.org/10.5772/intechopen.104167
Edited by Shailendra K. Saxena

Contributors
Yan Yan, Renfang Chen, Fábio A. Abade dos Santos, Teresa Fagulha, Sílvia S. Barros, Margarida Henriques, Ana Duarte, Fernanda Ramos, Tiago Luís, Margarida D. Duarte, Kollanoor Riji John, Mulloorpeedikayil Rosalind George, Panchavarnam Sivasankar, Abdulkarim F. Alhetheel, Faisal A. Alhetheel, Aishwarya Khamari, Akshya Kumar Mishra, Jijnasa Panda, Ratikanta Rath, Monika Khamari, Debashish Gardia, Kirti Nirmal, Seema Gangar, Shailendra K. Saxena, Supriya Shukla, Swatantra Kumar, Vimal K. Maurya, Saniya Ansari

First published in London, United Kingdom, 2023 by IntechOpen
IntechOpen is the global imprint of INTECHOPEN LIMITED, registered in England and Wales, registration number: 11086078, 5 Princes Gate Court, London, SW7 2QJ, United Kingdom

British Library Cataloguing-in-Publication Data
A catalogue record for this book is available from the British Library

Additional hard and PDF copies can be obtained from orders@intechopen.com

Viral Outbreaks - Global Impact and Newer Horizons
Edited by Shailendra K. Saxena
p. cm.
Print ISBN 978-1-83768-164-8
Online ISBN 978-1-83768-165-5
eBook (PDF) ISBN 978-1-83768-166-2

For EU product safety concerns:
IN TECH d.o.o., Prolaz Marije Krucifikse Kozulić 3, 51000 Rijeka, Croatia,
info@intechopen.com or visit our website at intechopen.com.

Meet the editor

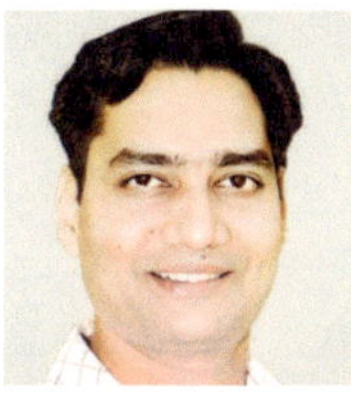

Professor Dr. Shailendra K. Saxena is a vice dean and professor at King George's Medical University, Lucknow, India. His research interests involve understanding the molecular mechanisms of host defense during human viral infections and developing new predictive, preventive, and therapeutic strategies for them using Japanese encephalitis virus (JEV), HIV, and emerging viruses as a model via stem cell and cell culture technologies. His research work has been published in various high-impact-factor journals. He has received many awards and honors in India and abroad, including various Young Scientist Awards, BBSRC India Partnering Award, and Dr. JC Bose National Award of the Department of Biotechnology, Min. of Science and Technology, Govt. of India. Dr. Saxena is a fellow of various prestigious international societies/academies including the Royal College of Pathologists, United Kingdom; Royal Society of Medicine, London; Royal Society of Biology, United Kingdom; Royal Society of Chemistry, London; and Academy of Translational Medicine Professionals, Austria. He was named a Global Leader in Science by *The Scientist*. He is also an international opinion leader/expert in the vaccination for Japanese encephalitis by IPIC (International Primary Immunodeficiency Congress) (UK).

Contents

Dedication

Dedicated
to my parents and family
who believed in academics
as the way forward for an intelligent mind
and
to the teachers
who introduced me to the subject
and nurtured my interest in it.

Preface

In the 21st century, the world has witnessed several waves of severe viral infectious disease outbreaks, including but not limited to the COVID-19 pandemic. Viral outbreaks are the major cause of infectious disease burden, placing substantial economic pressure on countries with low and lower-middle incomes. Rapid progress in urbanization in these countries and increased population density have created newer prospects of viral outbreaks and transmissions. Therefore, understanding the global spatial and temporal dispersal of newer viruses as well as the challenges that come along with them is vitally important.

Viral Outbreaks - Global Impact and Newer Horizons provides a comprehensive overview of the major viral global outbreaks. It discusses epidemiology, immunopathogenesis, viral genomics, diagnostic approaches, and antiviral pharmacology to combat these viral infections. This book is a useful resource for academics, policymakers, researchers, and students.

I wish to acknowledge all the authors for their valuable contributions. My research fellows and students are central to all my research and academic work. They are the motivating force behind anything constructive I do. They are truly brilliant and have a bright future. I would like to express my gratitude to my mentors, teachers, and students. I would also like to thank my colleagues, family, and friends who offered encouragement and support during my work on this book. A happy environment at home is essential for any kind of growth, and I thank my family, especially my wife and children, for the same.

Dr. Shailendra K. Saxena
Professor,
Center for Advanced Research (CFAR),
Faculty of Medicine,
King George's Medical University (KGMU),
Lucknow, India

Section 1

Viral Outbreaks: Global Trends

Chapter 1

Introductory Chapter: Recent Trends in Emerging and Reemerging Viral Contagions – The Day after Today

Shailendra K. Saxena, Supriya Shukla, Swatantra Kumar, Vimal K. Maurya and Saniya Ansari

1. Introduction

The increased interactions between people and animals and the easier spread of zoonotic pathogens have resulted from increased trade between communities. Following that, the emergence and spread of infectious diseases were facilitated by the growth of cities, the expansion of trade routes, increased travel, and the effects of an expanding human population on ecosystems, which increased the likelihood of outbreaks, epidemics, and even pandemics [1]. The terms "outbreak," "epidemic," and "pandemic" refer to a condition's occurrence in comparison to its expected rate as well as its geographic spread. An outbreak is defined as an unexpected rise in the population with a particular health condition or the occurrence of cases in a new location. An outbreak that spreads to a wider geographic area is called an epidemic. An epidemic that spreads globally is called a pandemic [2].

According to estimates, two-thirds of emerging human infections and about 60% of infectious diseases have zoonotic origins, with origins in wildlife. Humans are at high risk of infection as they are more likely to come into contact with animal and arthropod vectors of viral infections due to habitat destruction brought on by rapid urbanization. In the absence of specific immunity in these populations, such interactions have been one of the major factors increasing human susceptibility to infections by novel outbreaks [3]. Viral infections are majorly divided into three categories that are respiratory viral infections, arboviral infections, and bat-borne viral infections [4].

Over four million people die from acute respiratory diseases each year, and millions more are hospitalized in developing nations [5]. Human respiratory infections are brought on by more than 200 viral pathogens from the families *Orthomyxoviridae, Paramyxoviridae, Picornaviridae, Coronaviridae, Adenoviridae,* and *Herpesviridae*. Adenoviruses, Respiratory syncytial virus (RSV), influenza, and parainfluenza are still significant respiratory pathogens [6]. A recurring pattern in the world's landscape of infectious diseases has been the periods of dormancy that several pathogens experience after being first discovered, which are then preceded by their recurrence, frequently in more virulent forms. Arboviral diseases are transmitted by mosquitoes and are tedious to be diagnosed. The viral infections that are of major global concern are caused by arboviruses like West Nile virus (WNV), Japanese encephalitis virus (JEV), Dengue

IntechOpen

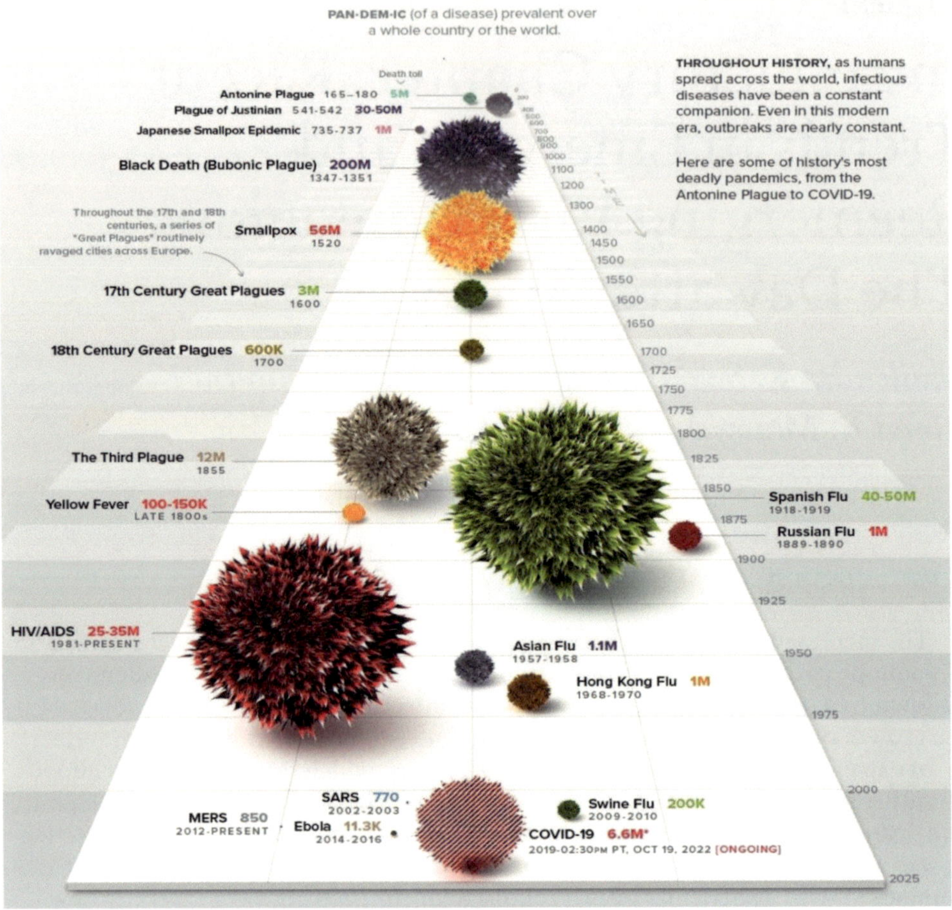
PAN·DEM·IC (of a disease) prevalent over a whole country or the world.
THROUGHOUT HISTORY, as humans spread across the world, infectious diseases have been a constant companion. Even in this modern era, outbreaks are nearly constant.
Here are some of history's most deadly pandemics, from the Antonine Plague to COVID-19.
Death toll
Antonine Plague 165–180 5M
Plague of Justinian 541-542 30-50M
Japanese Smallpox Epidemic 735-737 1M
Black Death (Bubonic Plague) 200M 1347-1351
Throughout the 17th and 18th centuries, a series of "Great Plagues" routinely ravaged cities across Europe.
Smallpox 56M 1520
17th Century Great Plagues 3M 1600
18th Century Great Plagues 600K 1700
The Third Plague 12M 1855
Yellow Fever 100-150K LATE 1800s
Spanish Flu 40-50M 1918-1919
Russian Flu 1M 1889-1890
HIV/AIDS 25-35M 1981-PRESENT
Asian Flu 1.1M 1957-1958
Hong Kong Flu 1M 1968-1970
SARS 770 2002-2003
MERS 850 2012-PRESENT
Ebola 11.3K 2014-2016
Swine Flu 200K 2009-2010
COVID-19 6.6M* 2019-02:30PM PT, OCT 19, 2022 [ONGOING]
1000
1100
1200
1300
1400
1450
1500
1550
1600
1650
1700
1725
1750
1775
1800
1825
1850
1875
1900
1925
1950
1975
2000
2025

Figure 1.
Visualizing the history of pandemics. Data sources: CDC, WHO, BBC, Wikipedia, Historical records, Encyclopaedia Britannica, Johns Hopkins University; Source: Visual Capitalist. https://www.visualcapitalist.com/history-of-pandemics-deadliest/.

virus (DENV), Chikungunya virus (CHIKV), Zika virus (ZIKV), Yellow fever virus (YFV), and others. *Aedes aegypti* mosquito populations are abundant throughout most of the nation, serving as effective carriers of DENV, CHIKV and ZIKV, which are still major threats worldwide (**Figure 1**, **Table 1**) [7].

2. Global outbreaks/pandemics in 21st century

2.1 Avian influenza

Humans can develop a variety of symptoms from asymptomatic or mild upper respiratory infections (fever and cough) to severe pneumonia, acute respiratory distress syndrome, shock, and even death from zoonotic influenza infections. The majority of human cases of avian influenza are brought on by direct or indirect contact with infected live or dead poultry or contaminated environments [8]. A total of 868 human cases of influenza A (H5N1) infection and 456 fatalities have been reported

Disease name	Time period	Causative agent	Deaths	CFR%
Global outbreaks/pandemics in 21st century				
Monkey pox	2022 onward	Monkeypox virus	51	3–6%
COVID-19	2019 onwards	Coronavirus	6.6 M	10%
Ebola	2014–2016	Ebolavirus	11,000	50%
MERS	2012 onwards	Coronavirus	858	34%
Swine flu	2009–2010	Influenza A virus subtype H1N1	2,00,000	0.40%
SARS	2002–2003	Coronavirus	770	9–11%
Global outbreaks/pandemics before 21st century				
Nipah	1999	Nipah Virus	265	40–75%
HIV/AIDS	1981 onwards	Human Immunodeficiency Virus	25–35 M	80%
Hong Kong Flu	1968–1970	Influenza A virus subtype H3N2	1 M	<1%
Asian Flu	1957–1958	Influenza A virus subtype H2N2	1.1 M	<2%
Spanish Flu	1918–1919	Influenza A virus subtype H1N1	40–50 M	2%
Russian Flu	1889–1890	Influenza A virus subtype H2N2	1 M	0.15%
Yellow Fever	Late 1800	Yellow Fever virus	100,000–150,000	39%
New World Smallpox	1520	Variola major virus	56 M	~1%
Japanese smallpox epidemic	735–737	Variola major virus	1 M	-
Antonine Plague	165–180	Believed to be either smallpox virus or measles virus	5 M	-

Table 1.
Global outbreaks/pandemics in and before 21st century.

globally from 21 countries between 2003 and October 21, 2022. Three human cases of influenza A (H5N1) infection have been reported in Europe thus far, including one case from the United Kingdom in 2021 and two cases from Spain in 2022 [9].

The average incubation time for the Influenza A (H5N1) virus is 2–5 days, but it can last up to 17 days. Humans who are infected typically experience fever, malaise, coughing, sore throats, and muscle aches. A pneumonia complication may cause severe illness and even death. In comparison to seasonal influenza infection, the case fatality rate for avian influenza in humans is significantly higher [10].

2.2 Ebola virus disease

The Sudan Ebolavirus (SUDV)-caused Ebola outbreak in the Republic of Uganda was declared on September 20, 2022, following the confirmation of a case in a village in Madudu Sub-County, Mubende District, central Uganda, on September 19 [11, 12]. Humans occasionally contract the severe, frequently fatal disease known as the Ebola virus disease (EVD), formerly known as Ebola hemorrhagic fever. The virus spreads among humans through human-to-human contact and also via animals. Around 50% of EVD cases end in death on average. In previous outbreaks, case fatality rates ranged from 25 to 90% [13].

Ebola vaccines have been designed and used to prevent the spread of outbreaks of the disease in Guinea and the Democratic Republic of the Congo (DRC). Infected individuals may be treated with early supportive care combined with early symptomatic treatment and re-hydration increases their survival. Inmazeb and Ebanga, two monoclonal antibodies, were authorized by the US Food and Drug Administration in late 2020 for the treatment of Zaire Ebola virus (Ebola virus) infection in adults and children [14].

2.3 Marburg virus disease

Marburg virus disease (MVD), formerly known as Marburg hemorrhagic fever, is a serious, often fatal illness that affects humans. It is a member of the same pathogen family as the Ebola virus. Due to two significant outbreaks that occurred concurrently in Marburg, Frankfurt, Belgrade, Serbia, as well as in Germany, the disease was first discovered in 1967 [15]. After nearly 18 years, two cases of Marburg virus disease were identified in Ghana's Ashanti region in July 2022. The risk of this 2022 outbreak spreading is high at the national level but low at the global level, according to WHO. The average fatality rate is around 50% in MVD cases. In previous outbreaks, case fatality rates ranged from 24 to 88%, depending on virus strain and case management [16].

The Fruit bats of the *Pteropodidae* family, *Rousettus aegyptiacus*, are thought to be natural hosts of the Marburg virus. The Marburg virus is transmitted to humans by fruit bats and spreads via human-to-human transmission [17]. Marburg virus infection is characterized by the sudden onset illness with excruciating headaches, high fever, and excruciating malaise. Within a week, many patients experience severe hemorrhagic symptoms, and in fatal cases, bleeding is typically present, frequently in multiple locations [15]. Early supportive care, including rehydration and symptom relief, improves survival. There is currently no licensed treatment that has been proven to neutralize the virus, but a variety of blood products, immune therapies, and drug therapies are being developed [18].

2.4 Yellow fever

A family of positive, single-stranded, enveloped RNA viruses known as the *Flaviviridae*. They can occasionally infect humans and are found in arthropods, primarily in ticks and mosquitoes [19]. The members of this family are major global causes of morbidity and mortality. YFV, DENV, JEV, WNV and ZIKV are a few of the viruses spread by mosquitoes [20].

Yellow fever is a viral hemorrhagic fever disease, transmitted by Aedes mosquitoes. Tropical regions of Africa, Central and South America are affected by this disease [21]. YF exhibits acute-onset jaundice along with constitutional symptoms like fatigue, headache, nausea, nausea, myalgia, fever, and nausea. Cases with severe symptoms may experience liver and multiple organ failure, and the CFR in these situations may reach 50% [22].

The IgM ELISA assay and qRT-PCR are the two main methods used in laboratory diagnosis. Due to the cross-reactivity with other flaviviruses, a plaque reduction neutralization test (PRNT) may be required. There is a YF vaccine that is incredibly effective. Within 10 days of vaccination (80–100% effective), and within 30 days (99% effective), a single dose of the YF vaccine is sufficient to confer life-long immunity [23]. An unprecedented initiative, the eliminate yellow fever epidemics (EYE) strategy was introduced in 2017. The EYE partnership with more than 50 partners assists 40 at-risk nations in Africa and the Americas in preventing, detecting, and responding to suspected cases and outbreaks of yellow fever. The collaboration aims to safeguard vulnerable populations, stop the global spread, and swiftly contain outbreaks. More than a billion people are anticipated to be immune to the illness by 2026 [24].

Zika virus was first discovered in Uganda in 1947 in monkeys. Later, in 1952, it was discovered in people in the United Republic of Tanzania and Uganda. The Island of Yap (Federated States of Micronesia) reported the first known outbreak of the zika virus disease in 2007. This was followed by a significant zika virus infection outbreak in 2013 in French Polynesia and other Pacific region nations and territories [25]. Other important mosquito-borne flaviviruses are Japanese encephalitis virus (JEV), is responsible for causing 68,000 clinical cases per year, which is the primary cause of viral encephalitis in many Asian nations. JEV transmission is endemic in 24 countries in the WHO South-East Asia and Western Pacific regions, putting the health of more than three billion people at risk [26].

2.5 Severe acute respiratory syndrome-associated coronavirus (SARS-CoV)

The SARS-associated coronavirus (SARS-CoV)causes respiratory disease known as a severe acute respiratory syndrome (SARS). It was discovered at the end of February 2003 as part of an outbreak that began in China and spread to four other countries [27]. SARS is an airborne virus that, like the common cold and influenza, can spread through small droplets of saliva. It was the first severe and easily transmissible new disease to emerge in the twenty-first century, with a clear capacity to spread along international air travel routes [28]. The majority of SARS patients were previously healthy adults aged 25–70 years. A few suspected SARS cases among children under the age of 15 have been reported. The case fatality rate among people is around 3% [29].

2.6 Nipah virus

In 1998, a case outbreak of acute febrile encephalitis among pig handlers in Kampung Sungai Nipah, Malaysia, led to the discovery of NiV for the first time. Nipah virus (NiV) is a pathogenic Paramyxovirus that, along with the Hendra virus, is a member of the Paramyxoviridae, genus Henipavirus. It causes acute-onset encephalitis, which can be fatal to humans [30]. Pteropus Bats are thought to be the reservoir for the NiV, and contact with positive NiV cases or an intermediate animal host, such as pigs, usually results in transmission to humans. The virus can also spread from person to person, according to reports [31]. There have been NiV outbreaks in pigs reported from Malaysia and Singapore. Human disease has since been reported in Bangladesh, India, Malaysia, and Singapore. The latest outbreak was seen in May 2018 in Kerala, India [32].

The average incubation period for NiV disease in humans is 4–14 days, while the maximum incubation period is 21 days. Acute febrile encephalitis is the condition that the virus causes and symptoms include fever, headache, drowsiness, dizziness, and coma. NiV infection in humans and animals is confirmed by anti-Nipah IgM and IgG antibody detection, virus isolation, and RNA analysis [33].

3. Global outbreaks that lead to Pandemic

3.1 Monkeypox

A viral zoonotic disease called monkeypox is most common in tropical rain-forest regions of Central and West Africa, with sporadic exportations to other areas. As of November 8, 2022, a total of 78,599 cases were reported in newer areas; where monkeypox has never been previously reported; while 949 cases were reported from the endemic area [34]. The Monkeypox virus, a species of the *Orthopoxvirus* genus in the family *Poxviridae*, is the culprit behind monkeypox. Typically, monkeypox is a self-limiting illness with symptoms that last between 2 and 4 weeks. There may be severe cases. The case fatality rate has recently been in the range of 3–6%. Humans can contract monkeypox by coming into close contact with an animal or person who has the disease, as well as by coming into contact with contaminated objects. By coming into close contact with lesions, bodily fluids, respiratory droplets, and contaminated objects like bedding, the monkeypox virus can spread from one person to another [35]. Clinical symptoms of monkeypox typically include fever, rash, and swollen lymph nodes, and it can result in a variety of health issues. The monkeypox vaccines used in the smallpox eradication program also offered protection from that disease. There are more recent vaccines available, one of which is authorized for the prevention of monkeypox [36].

3.2 SARS-CoV-2

Hospitals in Wuhan, Hubei province, China, reported on a cluster of pneumonia cases with no known cause on December 31, 2019, grabbing the attention of people all over the world. A new coronavirus was identified and named as Severe acute respiratory syndrome coronavirus 2 (SARS-CoV-2) which was identified 2 weeks later in a bronchioalveolar lavage of the patients. The SARS-CoV-2 causes respiratory infections along with multi-organ involvement disease known as Coronavirus disease (COVID-19) [37].

Over 627 million cases, including over 6.5 million fatalities, had been reported globally as of October 30, 2022 [38]. Both symptomatic and asymptomatic individuals can spread the virus to others by coming into close contact (within six feet) and exchanging respiratory droplets. Transmission may also happen through aerosols and possibly through contact with infected surfaces [39].

Due to the rapid emergence of some variants in populations and the evidence of transmission or clinical implications, these variants are regarded as variants of concern. Omicron (B.1.1.529) variants found in changing sub-lineages have dominated the world's circulating variants since 2022. At the same time, the Alpha (B.1.1.7), Beta (B.1.351), Gamma (P.1), and Delta (B.1.617.2) were prior variants of concern that are less circulating [40].

3.3 Influenza

The *Orthomyxoviridae* family of influenza viruses is frequently held responsible for epidemics and pandemics that affect humans. Prior to the 2009 pandemic, influenza pandemics occurred in 1918 (swine flu), 1957 (Asian flu), 1968 (Hong Kong flu), and 1977 (Russian flu) (pandemic influenza A H1N1) [41]. The influenza A, B, and C viruses are responsible for the acute respiratory illness influenza, which can appear locally or as a seasonal epidemic. Seasonal epidemics are brought on by the influenza A and B viruses, whereas influenza C viruses typically only cause minor illness. The antigenic characteristics of the two surface glycoproteins on influenza A viruses—hemagglutinin and neuraminidase—are used to further categorize them into subtypes. The influenza A virus has 16 hemagglutinin and 9 neuraminidase subtypes that have been isolated from birds (H1 to H16 and N1 to N9), and the RNA of an additional 2 haemagglutinin and neuraminidase subtypes that have been identified in bats (H17 and H18 and N10 and N11) [42].

The majority of human cases of avian influenza are brought on by direct or indirect contact with infected live or dead poultry or contaminated environments. A total of 868 human cases of influenza A (H5N1) infection, including these 2 cases, and 456 fatalities have been reported globally from 21 countries between 2003 and October 21, 2022. Three human cases of influenza A (H5N1) infection have been reported in Europe thus far, including one case from the United Kingdom in 2021 and two cases from Spain in 2022 [43].

Humans can develop a variety of symptoms from asymptomatic or mild upper respiratory infections (fever and cough) to severe pneumonia, acute respiratory distress syndrome, shock, and even death from zoonotic influenza infections. Animal influenza viruses can infect humans directly, and the resulting clinical illness can range from mild to severe, just like human influenza viruses [44]. A history of exposure to sick birds or travel to countries where avian influenza cases are being reported may raise suspicion of a novel influenza virus infection, but a definitive diagnosis requires laboratory tests that are typically only available through public health laboratories [9]. Identification of such infections is critical for determining the source of the virus, establishing evidence of person-to-person transmission, and assessing pandemic potential [41].

3.4 MERS-CoV

The zoonotic virus MERS-CoV, which causes respiratory infections, was first discovered in Saudi Arabia in 2012 and has since spread to 26 other nations. MERS-CoV infection has been linked to over 2207 lab-confirmed cases and 787 fatalities worldwide since 2012. The MERS-CoV clinical spectrum of illness includes asymptomatic infections all the way up to acute respiratory distress syndrome, which can lead to multiple organ failure and death. At 3–4 per 10 cases shows severe symptoms, the case-fatality rates (CFRs) have remained high [45].

The dynamics of this virus' transmission are currently poorly understood, and there is still no effective cure or preventative vaccine. Even in the absence of mutations conferring hyper-virulence, there is evidence for secondary, tertiary, and quaternary cases of MERS resulting from a single infected patient [46]. The natural reservoirs of this virus are bats, and patients have been reported who developed an infection from camels. The virus was transmitted in several countries' healthcare facilities, including transmission from patients to healthcare providers and transmission between patients before MERS-CoV was identified. Because symptoms and other clinical features may be nonspecific, it is not always possible to identify patients with MERS-CoV early or without testing [47].

4. Conclusions

The diversity in geo-climate of the world faces constant threat of viral outbreaks. It is impossible to predict when the next viral outbreak will start or what virus it will be. Therefore, non-pharmaceutical interventions should be used first to control the viral transmission from person to person, according to pandemic preparedness plans. For outbreaks to be successfully controlled, community involvement is essential. A combination of interventions, including case management, infection prevention and control procedures, surveillance and contact tracing, a top-notch laboratory service, safe and respectable burials, and social mobilization, are necessary for effective outbreak control.

5. Future perspectives

Disturbingly, future outbreaks and a pandemic are still a possibility because there are no vaccines for the various viral infectious strains, no effective treatments, and a high mortality rate. Therefore, it is crucial to ponder quickly about the disease and ways to stop a virus-related pandemic. There is a need for the creation of antivirals that are particular to the virus as well as vaccines against viral strains. All governments should make sure that their citizens have access to viral disease treatments. Additionally, for the prevention of viral transmission to the globe, it must be limited at the initial stage. To stop a future outbreak and potential pandemic, it is crucial to spread awareness early among people around the world.

Acknowledgements

The authors are grateful to the Vice Chancellor, King George's Medical University (KGMU) Lucknow, for the encouragement and support for this work. The authors have no other relevant affiliations or financial involvement with any organization or entity with a financial interest in or financial conflict with the subject matter or materials discussed in the manuscript apart from those disclosed.

Funding

This research did not receive any specific grant from funding agencies in the public, commercial, or not-for-profit sectors.

Conflict of interest

None.

Author details

Shailendra K. Saxena*, Supriya Shukla, Swatantra Kumar, Vimal K. Maurya and Saniya Ansari
Centre for Advanced Research (CFAR), Faculty of Medicine, King George's Medical University (KGMU), Lucknow, India

*Address all correspondence to: shailen@kgmcindia.edu

References

[1] Lindahl JF, Grace D. The consequences of human actions on risks for infectious diseases: A review. Infection Ecology & Epidemiology. 2015;**5**:30048. DOI: 10.3402/iee.v5.30048

[2] Grennan D. What is a pandemic? *JAMA*. 2019;**321**(9):910. DOI: 10.1001/jama.2019.0700

[3] World Health Organization. Asia Pacific strategy for emerging diseases 2005. Available from: https://apps.who.int/iris/handle/10665/204797. [Accessed: November 14, 2022]

[4] Gopalakrishnan R, Sureshkumar D, Thirunarayan MA, Ramasubramanian V. Melioidosis: An emerging infection in India. The Journal of the Association of Physicians of India. 2013;**61**(9):612-614

[5] Rao BL. Epidemiology and control of influenza. National Medical Journal of India. 2003;**16**(3):143-149

[6] Yezli S, Otter JA. Minimum infective dose of the major human respiratory and enteric viruses transmitted through food and the environment. Food and Environmental Virology. 2011;**3**(1):1-30. DOI: 10.1007/s12560-011-9056-7

[7] Paixão ES, Teixeira MG, Rodrigues LC. Zika, chikungunya and dengue: The causes and threats of new and re-emerging arboviral diseases. BMJ Global Health. 2018;**3**(Suppl. 1):e000530. DOI: 10.1136/bmjgh-2017-000530

[8] Uyeki TM, Hui DS, Zambon M, Wentworth DE, Monto AS. Influenza. Lancet. 2022;**400**(10353):693-706. DOI: 10.1016/S0140-6736(22)00982-5

[9] Poovorawan Y, Pyungporn S, Prachayangprecha S, Makkoch J. Global alert to avian influenza virus infection: From H5N1 to H7N9. Pathogens and Global Health. 2013;**107**(5):217-223. DOI: 10.1179/2047773213Y.0000000103

[10] Rothberg MB, Haessler SD, Brown RB. Complications of viral influenza. The American Journal of Medicine. 2008;**121**(4):258-264. DOI: 10.1016/j.amjmed.2007.10.040

[11] World Health Organization. Disease outbreak news (DONs) 2022. Available from: https://www.who.int/emergencies/disease-outbreak-news/item/2022-DON420. [Accessed: November 8, 2022]

[12] World Health Organization. Ebola disease caused by Sudan virus, Uganda 2022. Available from: https://www.who.int/emergencies/disease-outbreak-news/item/2022. [Accessed: November 10, 2022]

[13] To KK, Chan JF, Tsang AK, Cheng VC, Yuen KY. Ebola virus disease: A highly fatal infectious disease reemerging in West Africa. Microbes and Infection. 2015;**17**(2):84-97. DOI: 10.1016/j.micinf.2014.11.007

[14] Sivanandy P, Jun PH, Man LW, Wei NS, Mun NFK, Yii CAJ, et al. A systematic review of Ebola virus disease outbreaks and an analysis of the efficacy and safety of newer drugs approved for the treatment of Ebola virus disease by the US Food and Drug Administration from 2016 to 2020. Journal of Infection and Public Health. 2022;**15**(3):285-292. DOI: 10.1016/j.jiph.2022.01.005

[15] World health organization. Marburg virus disease 2021– factsheet Available from: https://www.who.int/news-room/fact-sheets/detail/marburg-virus-disease. [Accessed: November 9, 2022]

[16] Araf Y, Maliha ST, Zhai J, Zheng C. Marburg virus outbreak in 2022: A public health concern. The Lancet Microbe. 2022;**S2666-5247**(22):00258-0. DOI: 10.1016/S2666-5247(22)00258-0

[17] Sah R, Mohanty A, Reda A, Siddiq A, Mohapatra RK, Dhama K. Marburg virus re-emerged in 2022: Recently detected in Ghana, another zoonotic pathogen coming up amid rising cases of monkeypox and ongoing COVID-19 pandemic-global health concerns and counteracting measures. The Veterinary Quarterly. 2022;**42**(1):167-171. DOI: 10.1080/01652176.2022.2116501

[18] van Griensven J, De Weiggheleire A, Delamou A, Smith PG, Edwards T, Vandekerckhove P, et al. The use of Ebola convalescent plasma to treat Ebola virus disease in resource-constrained settings: A perspective from the field. *Clinical Infectious Diseases*. 2016;**62**(1):69-74. DOI: 10.1093/cid/civ680

[19] Centers for Disease Control and Prevention. Marburg outbreaks. 2022. Available from: https://www.cdc.gov/vhf/marburg/outbreaks/chronology.html [Accessed November 9, 2022]

[20] Centers for Disease Control and Prevention. Viral haemorrhage fever, flaviviridae 2022. Available from: https://www.cdc.gov/vhf/virus-families/flaviviridae.html. [Accessed November 9, 2022]

[21] Gardner CL, Ryman KD. Yellow fever: A reemerging threat. Clinics in Laboratory Medicine. 2010;**30**(1):237-260. DOI: 10.1016/j.cll.2010.01.001

[22] Isa SE, Onyedibe KI, Okolo MO, Abiba AE, Mafuka JS, Simji GS, et al. A 21-year-old student with fever and profound jaundice. *PLoS Neglected Tropical Diseases*. 2014;**8**(1):e2534. DOI: 10.1371/journal.pntd.0002534

[23] Domingo C, Charrel RN, Schmidt-Chanasit J, Zeller H, Reusken C. Yellow fever in the diagnostics laboratory. Emerging Microbes & Infections. 2018;**7**(1):129. DOI: 10.1038/s41426-018-0128-8

[24] World Health Organization. Yellow fever factsheet. 2018. Available from: https://www.who.int/news-room/fact-sheets/detail/yellow-fever. [Accessed: November 10, 2022]

[25] Kindhauser MK, Allen T, Frank V, Santhana RS, Dye C. Zika: The origin and spread of a mosquito-borne virus. Bulletin of the World Health Organization. 2016;**94**(9):675-686C. DOI: 10.2471/BLT.16.171082

[26] Suresh KP, Nayak A, Dhanze H, Bhavya AP, Shivamallu C, Achar RR, et al. Prevalence of Japanese encephalitis (JE) virus in mosquitoes and animals of the Asian continent: A systematic review and meta-analysis. Journal of Infection and Public Health. 2022;**15**(9):942-949. DOI: 10.1016/j.jiph.2022.07.010

[27] Xu RH, He JF, Evans MR, Peng GW, Field HE, Yu DW, et al. Epidemiologic clues to SARS origin in China. Emerging Infectious Diseases. 2004;**10**(6):1030-1037. DOI: 10.3201/eid1006.030852

[28] Zhu Z, Lian X, Su X, Wu W, Marraro GA, Zeng Y. From SARS and MERS to COVID-19: A brief summary and comparison of severe acute respiratory infections caused by three highly pathogenic human coronaviruses. Respiratory Research. 2020;**21**(1):224. DOI: 10.1186/s12931-020-01479-w

[29] World Health Organization. Disease outbreak news. 2022. Available from: www.who.int/emergencies/disease-outbreak-news/item/2022-DON420. [Accessed: November 10, 2022]

[30] Hauser N, Gushiken AC, Narayanan S, Kottilil S, Chua JV. Evolution of Nipah virus infection: Past, present, and future considerations. Tropical Medicine and Infectious Disease. 2021;**6**(1):24. DOI: 10.3390/tropicalmed6010024

[31] Kulkarni DD, Tosh C, Venkatesh G, Senthil KD. Nipah virus infection: Current scenario. Indian Journal of Virology. 2013;**24**(3):398-408. DOI: 10.1007/s13337-013-0171-y

[32] Sharma V, Kaushik S, Kumar R, Yadav JP, Kaushik S. Emerging trends of Nipah virus: A review. Reviews in Medical Virology. 2019;**29**(1):e2010. DOI: 10.1002/rmv.2010

[33] Mazzola LT, Kelly-Cirino C. Diagnostics for Nipah virus: A zoonotic pathogen endemic to Southeast Asia. BMJ Global Health. 2019;**4**(Suppl. 2):e001118. DOI: 10.1136/bmjgh-2018-001118

[34] Thornhill JP, Barkati S, Walmsley S, Rockstroh J, Antinori A, Harrison LB, et al. SHARE-net clinical group. Monkeypox virus infection in humans across 16 countries – April–June 2022. The New England Journal of Medicine. 2022;**387**(8):679-691. DOI: 10.1056/NEJMoa2207323

[35] Centers for Disease Control and Prevention. 2022 Monkeypox outbreak global map. 2022. Available from: https://www.cdc.gov/poxvirus/monkeypox/response/2022/world-map.html. [Accessed: November 14, 2022]

[36] Brooks JT, Marks P, Goldstein RH, Walensky RP. Intradermal vaccination for monkeypox - benefits for individual and public health. The New England Journal of Medicine. 2022;**387**(13):1151-1153. DOI: 10.1056/NEJMp2211311

[37] Wang C, Horby PW, Hayden FG, Gao GF. A novel coronavirus outbreak of global health concern. *Lancet* (London, England). 2020;**395**:470-473. DOI: 10.1016/s0140-6736 (20) 30185-9

[38] World Health Organization. Emergencies novel coronavirus 2019. 2022. Available from: https://www.who.int/emergencies/diseases/novel-coronavirus-2019. [Accessed November 10, 2022]

[39] Tang S, Mao Y, Jones RM, Tan Q, Ji JS, Li N, et al. Aerosol transmission of SARS-CoV-2? Evidence, prevention and control. Environment International. 2020;**144**:106039. DOI: 10.1016/j.envint.2020.106039

[40] Dhawan M, Saied AA, Mitra S, Alhumaydhi FA, Emran TB, Wilairatana P. Omicron variant (B.1.1.529) and its sublineages: What do we know so far amid the emergence of recombinant variants of SARS-CoV-2? Biomedicine & Pharmacotherapy. 2022;**154**:113522. DOI: 10.1016/j.biopha.2022.113522

[41] Paules C, Subbarao K. Influenza. *Lancet*. 2017;**390**(10095):697-708. DOI: 10.1016/S0140-6736(17)30129-0

[42] Tong S, Zhu X, Li Y, Shi M, Zhang J, Bourgeois M, et al. New world bats harbor diverse influenza A viruses. *PLoS Pathogens*. 2013;**9**(10):e1003657. DOI: 10.1371/journal.ppat.1003657

[43] Potdar V, Brijwal M, Lodha R, Yadav P, Jadhav S, Choudhary ML, et al. Identification of human case of avian influenza A(H5N1) infection, India. *Emerging Infectious Diseases*. 2022;**28**(6):1269-1273. DOI: 10.3201/eid2806.212246

[44] Sampath S, Khedr A, Qamar S, Tekin A, Singh R, Green R, et al. Pandemics throughout the history. *Cureus*. 2021;**13**(9):e18136. DOI: 10.7759/cureus.18136

[45] Mostafa A, Kandeil A, Shehata M, El Shesheny R, Samy AM, Kayali G, et al. Middle East Respiratory Syndrome Coronavirus (MERS-CoV): State of the Science. Microorganisms. 2020;**8**(7):991. DOI: 10.3390/microorganisms8070991

[46] Mourya DT, Yadav PD, Ullas PT, Bhardwaj SD, Sahay RR, Chadha MS, et al. Emerging/re-emerging viral diseases & new viruses on the Indian horizon. The Indian Journal of Medical Research. 2019;**149**(4):447-467. DOI: 10.4103/ijmr.IJMR_1239_18

[47] Cowling BJ, Park M, Fang VJ, Wu P, Leung GM, Wu JT. Preliminary epidemiological assessment of MERS-CoV outbreak in South Korea. Euro Surveillance. 2015;**20**(25):7-13. DOI: 10.2807/1560-7917.es2015.20.25.21163

Section 2

Viral Outbreaks Linked to Humans

Chapter 2

Rotaviral Diseases and Their Implications

Kirti Nirmal and Seema Gangar

Abstract

Rotaviruses (Latin rota, "wheel"), the name derived from the wheel-like appearance of the virions when viewed by negative-contrast electron microscopy Rotavirus, are one of the foremost causes of rigorous peadiatric diarrhea globally. According to WHO, it is the primary cause of severe diarrhea among young children, leading to 4.5 million hospitalizations and more than 700,000 deaths of children aged 5 and under annually. The viruses are present in the stool of an infected person and can remain viable for a long time on contaminated surfaces, including people's hands. They are transmitted by fecal-oral route. Fecal contamination of food and water are common reservoirs and fingers, flies and fomites play vehicular role in transmission of rotaviruses. Both symptomatic and asymptomatic infections can lead to viral transmission due to shedding of viruses, often observed in close contacts, day care centers or via infected food handlers or healthcare workers. The disease manifested the symptoms of rotavirus infection, which may last up to 8 days and comprises fever, nausea, vomiting, abdominal cramps, and frequent, watery diarrhea. Two types of the rotavirus vaccine RotaTeq (RV5) and Rotarix (RV1) are available. Both vaccines are administrated orally, not as a shot. This chapter focuses on new information related to the clinical presentation and pathogenesis of rotavirus infection and its implications.

Keywords: rotavirus, disease, virus, systematic review

1. Introduction

Rotaviruses are recognized as a major cause of viral gastroenteritis among children since 1973 when Ruth F. Bishop and his colleagues observed the virus particles in the duodenal epithelial cells of gastroenteritis patients by electron microscopy [1]. As per WHO, Rotaviruses are responsible for approximately 453,000 deaths/year among children aged <5 years, globally, and over 2 million children are hospitalized each year with pronounced dehydration from rotavirus infection [2].

2. Taxonomy

The rotavirus (RV) genome is comprised of eleven segments of double-stranded RNA (dsRNA) and is contained within a non-enveloped, icosahedral particle.

During assembly, a highly-coordinated selective packaging mechanism ensures that progeny RV virions contain one of each genome segment. It has two subfamilies: Sedoreovirinae and Spinareovirinae [3].

3. Morphology

The name Rotaviruses (Latin *rota*, "wheel") is derived from the wheel-like appearance of the virions when viewed by negative-contrast electron microscopy (**Figure 1**). The mature virion has an approximate diameter of about 100 nm and possesses icosahedral symmetry. It is made up of three concentric protein layers and thus also known as a "triple-layered particle" or TLP. The mature virion lacks a lipid envelope (**Figure 2**) [4]. However, there is the acquisition of a transient lipid envelope during the budding of immature particles into the endoplasmic reticulum (ER). The triple-layered capsid encloses 11 discrete segments (seg 1–11) of linear dsRNA, which codes for six structural viral proteins, (VP1, VP2, VP3, VP4, VP6, and VP7) and six non-structural viral proteins (NSP1-NSP6). Each segment of dsRNA codes one protein except for segment 11, which codes two proteins (**Figure 3**) [5].

The outermost layer of the capsid is an icosahedral-shaped lattice made up of 780 copies of VP7 (38 kDa), a glycoprotein, and 120 copies of the spike protein VP4 (88 kDa) [6]. As per cryo-EM studies, VP4 has a large globular domain that is buried inside the inner layer, and it forms the spikes that emanate through the outer layer, which helps in cell attachment, penetration, hemagglutination, neutralization, and virulence of Rotaviruses [7]. The VP4 or the spike protein has a trypsin cleavage site along its length. The infectivity of virus particles gets enhanced by several folds on proteolytic cleavage of VP4 (88 kDa) into VP8* (28 kDa) and VP5* (60 kDa). It induces conformational changes to stabilize the spike protein. VP8* and VP5* remain

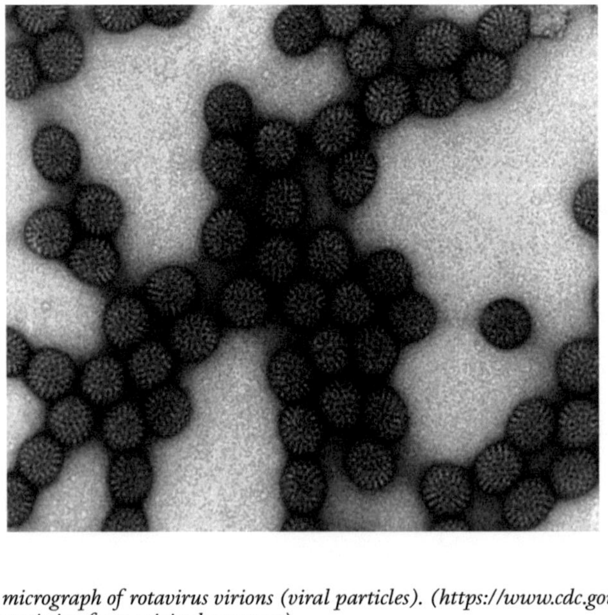

Figure 1.
Transmission electron micrograph of rotavirus virions (viral particles). (https://www.cdc.gov/rotavirus/about/photos.html) (taken permission from original resources).

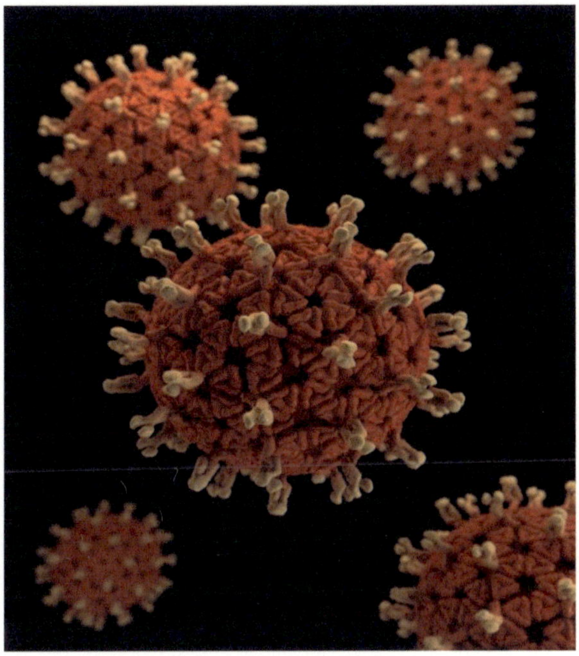

Figure 2.
3D graphical representation of rotavirus virions (viral particles). Rotavirus is known and named for the wheel-like appearance visible under an electron microscope (taken permission from original resources).

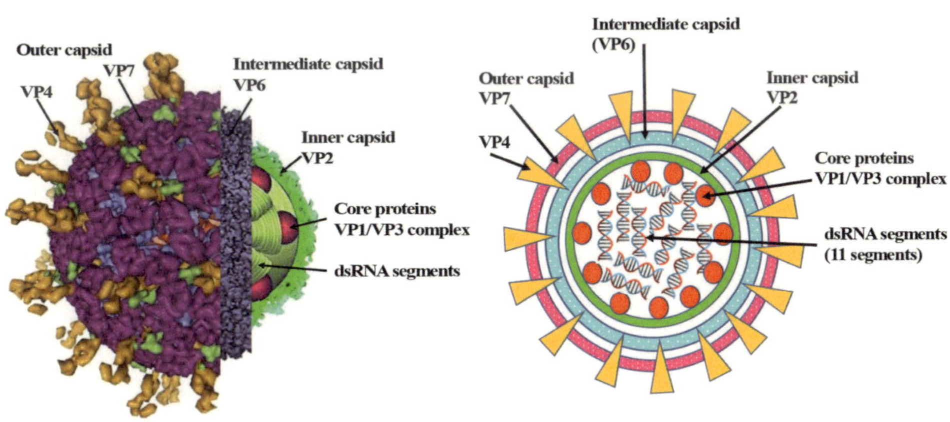

Figure 3.
Structure of rotavirus.

associated with the virion and facilitate virus entry into cells [8]. The intermediate layer of the virion is formed by 260 VP6 trimers in an icosahedral shape. The outer two layers consist of 132 aqueous channels of three types (types I–III), which play an important role in the transcription and translocation of mRNA. The virus particles that lack the outer layer are non-infectious and known as double-layered particles (DLPs), and particles that lack the outer two layers are known as single-layered particles (SLPs) [9]. The VP2 is the most abundant protein; it interacts with genomic

RNA on the inside and the VP6 layer on its outer side. The rest of the core proteins are present in small quantities and provide the enzymatic functions required for producing the capped mRNA transcripts [10]. The components of outermost layer (VP7 and VP4) carry epitopes for eliciting neutralizing antibodies independently. Based on this, a dual classification system was established decades ago to define Rotavirus G (VP7 is a **G**lycoprotein) and P (VP4 is **P**rotease sensitive) genotypes. So far, 36 G genotypes and 51 P serotypes have been identified [11].

4. Nucleic acid

The genome of rotaviruses consists of 11 discrete segments of linear dsRNA of 18,555 bp size. The size of the segments ranges from 667 bp to 3302 bp. The genome is A + U rich (58–67%). **Table 1** describes the size, protein products encoded by segments of dsRNA, and functions of proteins of the Rotaviruses group [5, 11]. The minor proteins VP1 and VP3 form a heterodimer, which is anchored to the inner surface (N-terminal residues) of the VP2 layer and is known as the transcription enzyme complex. The VP2 layer in addition to proper positioning of the transcription enzyme complex helps in the regulation of endogenous transcription of the genome [5, 12]. The transcription of the genome is a dynamic process, the dsRNA segments move around the anchored transcription enzyme complex (**Figure 3**). The similar assembly of the structures has been observed in members of ortho-reoviruses; however, their capping enzyme is outside the innermost layer (**Table 1**).

5. Replication

Rotaviruses enter the body via the fecal-oral route and infect the epithelial cells of the villi in the small intestine. The virus multiplies in the cytoplasm of the epithelial cells [12]. The rotaviruses replicate well in continuous cell cultures derived from monkey kidneys. The replication cycle is approximately completed in 12–15 h at 37°C. The replication cycle can be divided into the following steps (**Figure 4**) [8]. The following steps need to be followed for replication of the virus. Attachment (mediated by VP4 and VP7), Penetration and uncoating, Synthesis of the plus strand of ssRNA (which also acts as mRNA), Formation of viroplasm, RNA packaging, synthesis of minus-strand and DLP formation, and Virus particle maturation (TLP formation) and release.

5.1 Attachment

The VP4 or the spike protein is the viral attachment protein of the TLPs. The VP8* subunit of VP4 (at the tip of the spikes) interacts with the sialoglycans (such as gangliosides GM1 and GD1a) and non-sialoglycans receptors such as histo-blood group antigens (HBGAs), receptors present on the host cell [13, 14]. Several integrins ($\alpha2\beta$ 1, $\alpha\nu\beta3$, $\alpha x\beta2$, and $\alpha4\beta1$) and heat shock protein 70 (hsc70) serve as co-receptors, which interact with VP5* or VP7 [15]. The VP8* subunit also mediates hemagglutination in some strains of rotaviruses [10, 16]. The VP4 spike undergoes conformational change the moment it interacts with the host cell receptors leading

RNA segment no	Size (bp)	Protein encoded	Mol. mass of protein (kDa)	Function
1	3302	VP1 (RdRp)	125	RdRP; minor core component activated by VP2
2	2690	VP2	102.4	RNA binding activity; sub-group specificity antigen
3	2591	VP3 (cap)	98.1	Capping enzyme. Minor core component with guanylyltransferase, methyltransferase, 2′–5′ oligoadenylate phosphodiesterase and ssRNA binding activities
4	2362	VP4	86.8	Viral attachment spike protein activated by trypsin cleavage to generate 1. VP5* 60 kDa (membrane penetration) and 2. VP8* 28 kDa (carbohydrate binding, with haemaglutination activity) moieties. P-type neutralization antigen.
5	1611	NS53 NSP1 (VP5)	58.7	Putative viral E3 ubiquitin ligase, with RNA binding activity
6	1356	VP6	44.8	Trimeric protein major component of inner capsid. Group and sub-group specificity antigen.
7	1059	NSP3 (VP9)	34.6	Binds to viral mRNA and cellular eIF4G; promotes circularization of viral mRNAs; inhibits host translation
8	1104	NS35 NSP2 (VP8)	36.7	Essential viroplasm component that interacts with NSP5; forms viral inclusion body or viroplasm matrix protein. Octamer with NTPase, RTPase, ssRNA binding and helix destabilizing activities
9	1062	VP7 VP7 (cleaved form)	37.4 33.9	Virion surface glycoprotein, forming Ca^{2+}-stabilized trimer. G-type neutralization antigen
10	751	NSP4 (VP12)	20.3	RER transmembrane glycoprotein, binds DLPs, essential for budding into ER and addition of outer capsid, act as viral enterotoxin, disrupts Ca^{2+} homeostasis
11	667	NSP5 (VP11)	21.7	RNA binding activity; essential viroplasm component that interacts with NSP2
		NSP6	11	RNA binding activity. Interacts with NSP5; non-essential viroplasm component

Table 1.
The number of and size of each gene segment and the functions of their encoded proteins.

to the exposure of the VP5* subunit, which is normally hidden under VP8*. The trypsin facilitates this virus's entry into cells by inducing conformational changes and stabilizing the spike protein.

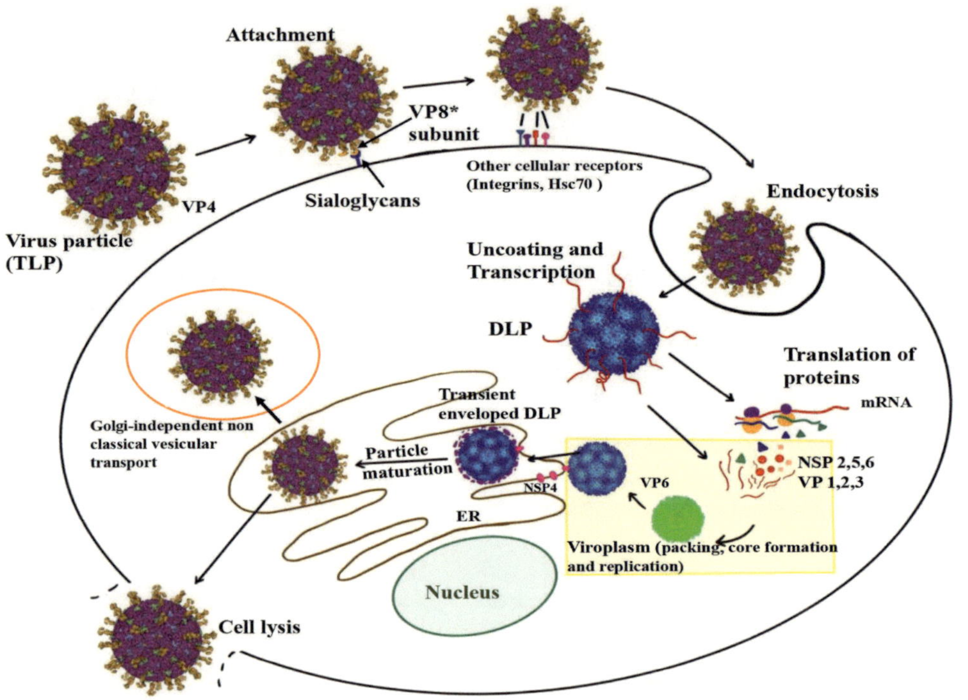

Figure 4.
The rotavirus replication cycle. The rotavirus triple-layered particles (TLPs) first attach to sialo-glycans on the host cell surface, followed by interactions with other cellular receptors (integrins and Hsc70). Virus is then internalized by receptor-mediated endocytosis. Removal of the outer layer, triggered by the low calcium of the endosome, results in the release of transcriptionally active double-layered particles (DLPs) into the cytoplasm. The DLPs start rounds of mRNA transcription, and these mRNAs are used to translate viral proteins. Once enough viral proteins are made, the RNA genome is replicated and packaged into newly made core in specialized structures called viroplasms. Addition of VP6 protein to the core forms the DLPs. The newly made DLPs bind to NSP4, which serves as an endoplasmic reticulum (ER) receptor, and bud into the ER. NSP4 also acts as a viroporin to release Ca^{2+} from intracellular stores. Transiently enveloped particles are seen in the ER. The transient membranes are removed as the outer capsid proteins VP4 and VP7 assemble, resulting in the maturation of the TLPs. The progeny virions are released through cell lysis.

5.2 Penetration and uncoating

After binding, the virusparticles (TLPs) penetrate the host cell either by receptor-mediated endocytosis or direct membrane penetration. Due to low Ca^{2+} concentrations in endosomes, the outer capsid proteins (VP4 and VP7) solubilize and release the transcriptionally active DLP form in the cytoplasm of the host cell [17].

5.3 Synthesis of the plus strand of ssRNA and viroplasm formation

The transcription complexes (RdRp/VP1/Capping enzymeVP3) in the core of the DLPs are complex with the dedicated segment of viral dsRNA [17, 18]. The negative strand of the genomic RNA acts as a template, and the transcription complex synthesizes a capped, non-polyadenylated plus (+) ssRNA, which is released in the cytoplasm via type I aqueous channels [18]. These plus (+) ssRNA transcripts serve two functions. First, they are used for the translation of virus-encoded proteins in the cytoplasm, thus also called mRNA, and later on in the replication cycle, they act as templates for negative-sense strand synthesis and producing dsRNA genome segments [16–18].

5.4 Formation of the viroplasm

Two non-structural proteins NSP2 and NSP5 mediate the synthesis of virion assembly in cytoplasmic inclusions termed viroplasms. NSP2 octamer forms a complex with VP1, VP2, and tubulin to form viroplasms. The NSP2 octamer has a binding site for which NSP5 and (+)ssRNA compete, thus it regulates the balance between translation and replication [19].

5.5 RNA packaging, synthesis of minus-strand RNA, and DLP formation

The transcription complex interacts with VP2 decamer, NSP5, and NSP2 and forms the core particle The 11 different (+) ssRNA segments interact with the transcription complex and VP2 and are then packaged [20]. This interaction leads to the synthesis of a negative-sense strand and results in the formation of cores containing a complete set of 11 dsRNA segments. Once formed, VP6 is added to the core leading to the synthesis of DLPs [20].

5.6 Virus particle maturation (TLP formation) and release

The NSP4 is a transmembrane glycoprotein, located in the endoplasmic reticulum (ER). It interacts with the VP6 protein and acts as an intracellular receptor for DLPs [21]. The NSP4 acts as viroporin as it increases intracellular Ca^{2+} levels by releasing Ca^{2+} from intracellular stores. The elevated levels of intracellular Ca^{2+} are needed to stabilize the outer layer of TLPs, and it activates a kinase-dependent pathway, which leads to autophagy [22]. NSP4 also acts as viral enterotoxin and interacts with non-infected intestinal cells [21, 22]. Interaction of NSP4 and DLP is crucial in the maturation process. The DLPs are recruited to the ER. Budding of DLPs through the ER results in the transient acquisition of a lipid envelope followed by the acquisition of the outermost layers by the addition of VP4 and VP7 to the DLPs. The newly formed TLPs are then released by either cell lysis or exocytosis [8].

5.7 Physical properties

The outermost layer (VP7 and VP4) of the infectious triple-layer particles (TLPs) can be destabilized with Ca^{2+}-chelating agents, such as EDTA, leading to the loss of the outermost layer and formation of double-layered particles (DLPs). The DPLs are non-infectious. The virion became non-infectious by treating it with 95% ethanol, 0.1% sodium dodecyl sulfate, beta-propiolactone, chlorine, formalin, and phenols. The hemagglutinin activity of VP4 is lost at 45°C or by freezing and thawing [4, 5].

6. Pathogenesis

Rotaviruses are ubiquitous, and TLPs are relatively stable in the environment. They are transmitted by the fecal-oral route. Fecal contamination of food and water are common reservoirs and fingers, flies and fomites play a vehicular role in the transmission of rotaviruses. Both symptomatic and asymptomatic infections can lead to viral transmission due to the shedding of viruses, often observed in close contact, with day care centers, or via infected food handlers or healthcare workers [23].

The rotaviruses mainly infect the villi of small intestinal mucosa leading to loss of microvilli, villous atrophy, and necrosis of the gut epithelium. The virions extensively replicate in the cytoplasm of enterocytes and damage their transport mechanism resulting in electrolytes and fluid malabsorption leading to increased osmotic pressure in the gut lumen and subsequently onset of diarrhea [8, 24].

The NSP4 protein, encoded by rotaviruses, is a viral enterotoxin that induces calcium ion-dependent chloride secretion into the intestinal lumen via activating signal transduction pathways through phospholipase C. The NSP4 inactivates the Sodium-Glucose-Lactose-Transporter proteins system (SGLT1) that mediates the reabsorption of water, sugar, and body electrolytes. The NSP4 also stimulates the enteric nervous system by inducing the secretion of serotonin (5-HT: 5-hydroxytryptamine) from enteroendocrine cells due to an increase in intracellular calcium concentration, thus increasing gut motility [24, 25].

7. Clinical manifestations

Rotaviruses are the major cause of diarrheal illness in infants and children worldwide. The infectious dose is low (<100 TLPs), and the incubation period is of 18–36 h followed by acute onset of symptoms. The symptoms vary from mild to severe watery diarrhea, vomiting, abdominal pain, fever, and dehydration. Diarrhea may last for

Virus morphology	The rotavirus belongs to the family Reoviridae. Only virus family to have dsRNA. There are six structural viral proteins (VP1 to VP7 except for VP5). VP 6 is group-specific.
Pathogenesis	Transmitted by the fecal-oral route, they destroy enterocytes of the small intestine; however gastric and colonic mucosa are spared. Non-structural protein- NSP4, acts as enterotoxin and induces secretion by altering epithelial cell function and permeability.
Clinical manifestations	In developing countries like India, Rotavirus illness occurs at a younger age. Incubation period: 1–3 days, Abrupt onset, characterized by vomiting, watery diarrhea, fever, and abdominal pain. Few children may suffer from severe loss of electrolytes and fluid leading to dehydration, while rest may recover. Adults are usually asymptomatic but show seroconversion.
Laboratory diagnosis	Direct detection of virus: Feces collected early in the illness is the most ideal specimen. It can be demonstrated in stool by: Immuno-electrophoresis microscopy: Sharp-edgedtriple-shelled capsid, looks like the spokes grouped around the hub of the wheel. Isolation of rotavirus is difficult. Detection of viral antigen: In stool by ELISA and Latex-agglutination based methods RT-PCR: is the most sensitive detection method for the detection of rotavirus from stool Typing method: G serotypes and P genotypes of rotaviruses can be detected by RNA sequence typing and neutralization test Serologic test: Can be done by ELISA to detect the rise of antibody titer.
General preventive measures	Measures to improve hygiene and sanitation in the community and contact precautions such as strict hand hygiene.
Prophylaxis	The WHO prequalified oral rotavirus vaccines introduction have yielded significant decline in global burden of rotavirus associated infections. These include four vaccines Rotavac, Rotarix; Rotateq and Rotasiil. All four vaccines are safe with good efficacy. Rotatac and Rotasiil are manufactured in India while others are manufactured outside India.

Table 2.
Summary of rotavirus.

5–7 days. The majority of patients usually recover completely. Infected adults are usually asymptomatic or rarely exhibit symptoms. However, infants and children may suffer because of severe loss of fluid and electrolytes leading to dehydration or death if untreated. The excretion of viruses in the stool may persist up to 50 days after the onset of diarrhea (**Table 2**).

8. Epidemiology

As per WHO, more than 25 million outpatient visits and more than 2 million hospitalizations each year globally are due to severe, dehydrating diarrhea by rotavirus infections in children aged less than 5 years. Generally, the mortality rate is higher in low and middle-income countries as compared with high-income countries. In low and middle-income countries, approximately 75% of children acquire their first episode of rotavirus infection within 12 months of age, whereas children of 2–5 years of age are predominantly infected in high-income countries. The group A rotaviruses (RVA) is the major group that accounts for more than 90% of rotavirus infections in humans worldwide [26]. Rotavirus gastroenteritis is predominantly seen during cool, dry seasons thus also known as "winter diarrhea" and in tropical areas, it can be seen all the year around [27]. Nosocomial outbreaks of rotaviruses are common in pediatric wards, elderly, and immunocompromised patients.

9. Lab diagnosis

A fresh stool sample should be collected in well-labeled, clean wide-mouth container for the presence of the virus, virus-specific antigen, or RNA by direct or indirect detection methods. Rectal swabs can also be taken, but they are not ideal samples [27].

9.1 Direct method

The demonstration of the viral particle in stool sample by electron microscopy shows a typical wheel-shaped virion. The sensitivity and specificity can be improved by immune-electron microscopy by adding specific antiviral antibodies to the specimen or by utilizing magnetic microparticles functionalized with monoclonal antibodies to enhance the ability to capture, concentrate, separate, and detect infectiously [28]. The rotavirus can be cultured on cell lines such as monkey kidney cell line to confirm viral viability and also improves the molecular detection of the virus in clinical samples where low viral load is present, although the method is highly sensitive, it is time-consuming, expensive, highly prone to contamination, and is usually available at research-based laboratories [20].

9.2 Indirect method

Indirect detection of viruses by a variety of molecular assays to detect antigens, antibodies, or viral RNA is more popular, cost-effective, and less time-consuming as compared with direct methods. Commercially available antigen detection kits based on various principles such as immunochromatography or latex agglutination are widely used point-of-care tests for rotavirus diagnosis in resource-limited nations.

The ELISA-based antigen detection techniques are the most widely recognized screening platform with high sensitivity and specificity. A large sample volume can be tested on a 96-well plate [28, 29]. Other immunoassays such as radioimmunoassay, counter-Immuno-electrophoresis, and fluorescent antibody staining are also used.

9.3 Molecular method

The detection of the rotaviral genome through polymerase chain reaction–based methods (e.g., RT-PCR, RT-qPCR, real-time PCR, and multiplex RT-PCR) are revolutionary as a research tool as well as for diagnosis. Newer PCR-based techniques such as RT-qPCR assays are more sensitive and specific than antigen detection and are suitable for genotyping and sequencing with faster turnaround time as compared with conventional methods [29].

10. Treatment

The treatment is mainly supportive and consists of rehydration by the oral or intravenous route to restore the loss of water and electrolytes. Commercial preparations of oral rehydration solution (ORS) are available over the counter. To restore the damaged mucosal epithelial lining, the ORS is supplemented with zinc tablets [30].

There is currently no antiviral drug approved for the treatment of rotavirus infections.

There have been studies that demonstrate the anti-rotavirus activity of some drugs such as Nitazoxanide (100 mg in 12–47 months and 200 mg in 4 years old, twice daily for consecutive 3 days) an oralsynthetic anti-parasitic agent inhibits viro plasma formation; gemcitabine, an anticancer drug, with pyrimidine nucleotide inhibitor activity inhibits rotavirus as well. Resveratrol (Inhibitor of viral protein synthesis), Ziyuglycoside II (Inhibitor of TLR4/NF-kB pathway), Brequinar (pyrimidine biosynthesis inhibitor), 2^0-*C*-methyl nucleosides (viral polymerase inhibitor), Racecadotril (Intestinal enkephalinase inhibitor, which suppresses the secretion of water and electrolytes into the gut), ML-60218 (RNA polymerase III inhibitors), and Genipin (Entry inhibitor) are potent antiviral drugs [31, 32].

11. Prevention

General preventive measures:

The rotavirus infection can be prevented by good hygiene measures such as personal hygiene mainly hand and sanitary. Maintenance of food safety standards, safe water supply, and environmental hygiene are essential in preventing outbreaks at food outlets. The WHO recommends continued breastfeeding as maternal antibodies have a protective role and help in reducing the duration and severity of diarrhea [33].

11.1 Rotavirus vaccine

The rotavirus vaccines that have been licensed by WHO are RotaTeq, Rotarix, Rotavac, and ROTASIIL for the prevention and control of rotavirus gastroenteritis

11.1.1 RotaTeq (RV5)

RotaTeq (RV5) is an oral live attenuated pentavalent vaccine developed by Merck and Co. Inc., USA, and approved by WHO in 2008. RotaTeq is given in three doses at ages 2 months, 4 months, and 6 months. It is a human-bovine reassorted live attenuated vaccine containing four human VP7(G) types (G1, G2, G3, and G4) and one human VP4(P) type. The efficacy of the vaccine in developed nations such as in European countries is higher at 98%; however, the efficacy reduces in low socioeconomic countries such as Asia at 51% and African countries at 64%. Multiple factors such as malnutrition, enteric co-infections, poor maternal health, prevalent strain diversity, and poor maintenance of cold chain storage lead to reduce effectiveness and efficacy of the vaccine in low socioeconomic countries [34, 35].

11.1.2 Rotarix (RV1)

Rotarix (RV1) is an oral live attenuated monovalent vaccine developed by GlaxoSmithKline Biologicals and approved by WHO in 2009. It is human rotavirus G1P8 genotype months for the prevention of rotavirus gastroenteritis caused by G1 and non-G1 types (G3, G4, and G9). The vaccine is available in lyophilized form, which can be stored at 2°–8°C. It should be used within 24 h of reconstitution in provided diluent. The vaccine is given in two doses (1 ml each) 4 weeks apart. The first dose should be administered before 15 weeks of age, and the two dose series should be completed before 8 months. Similar to RotaTeq, the efficacy reduces to 62–85% in developing countries as compared with developed countries (96%) [36].

11.1.3 Live attenuated, oral vaccine by Bharat Biotech, India, in 2018

Recently, WHO prequalified another live attenuated, oral vaccine by Bharat Biotech, India, in 2018. It is a monovalent liquid frozen vaccine containing wild-type reassortant G9P11 (116E) strain of rotavirus, prepared in Vero cells. The vaccine is administered as a 3-dose regimen, 4 weeks apart, beginning at 6 weeks of age. The vaccine should not be administered to children older than 8 months of age. The vaccine can be stored at 2–8°C for 7 for months and −20°C for long-term (5 years). The vaccine efficacy is 56.4% (37–70%) in the first year of life in developed countries [37, 38].

11.1.4 Rotasiil

Rotasiil, developed by the Serum Institute of India, is a pentavalent vaccine containing a lyophilized preparation of live attenuated human-bovine rotavirus reassortant G1, G2, G3, G4, and G9 strains. The vaccine is available in Lyophilized, Thermostable lyophilized and Liquid formulations and thus can be kept at <40°C for up to 18 months and <25°C for up to 30 months. The three doses are given at 6 weeks, 10 weeks, and 14 weeks [38].

11.1.5 Rotavin-M1 (POLYVAC, ThànhphË Hà NÎi, Vietnam) and Lanzhou lamb (Lanzhou Institute of biological product, China)

Recently, two vaccines have been licensed in Vietnam and India are Rotavin-M1 (POLYVAC, ThànhphË Hà NÎi, Vietnam) and Lanzhou lamb (Lanzhou Institute of biological product, China) respectively though yet to be licensed by WHO, and their coverage is limited [38].

11.1.6 Rotavin-M1

Rotavin-M1 is a live attenuated human rotavirus strain G1P8 available in the liquid frozen formulation, which can be stored 2–8°C for 2 months and 20°C for 24 months. Two doses are required minimum at 6 weeks of age, for 4 weeks apart. On the other hand, Lanzhou lamb is a live attenuated lamb G10P15 rotavirus strain available in the liquid formulation, which can be stored at 2–8°C for 12 months [37, 38]. The vaccine is given as a single dose followed by annual boosters for children aged between 2 months and 3 years [35]. Rotavirus causes acute gastroenteritis among children less than 5 years of age. Early detection and treatment are crucial to prevent mortality. Improvement in vaccination coverage, safe water supply, personal and environmental hygiene, continued surveillance, and knowledge of circulating genotypes of the virus in the environment are needed.

Rotavac and Rotasiil are manufactured in India, while others are manufactured outside India.

12. Conclusion

Rotavirus remains the leading cause of severe acute dehydrating diarrhea among infants and young children for four decades with a substantial effect on morbidity and mortality. This infection is primarily localized to the intestinal enterocytes leading to necrosis of mucosal cells by various mechanisms and subsequently secretory-driven watery diarrhea. It is to be expected that together with rotavirus-mediated gastroenteritis such extra-intestinal manifestations will become less prevalent as a consequence of the introduction of anti-rotavirus vaccination. Clinicians, particularly pediatricians caring for rotavirus-infected children, should be aware of the possible extra-intestinal complications of rotavirus infection. The currently available vaccines have significantly reduced mortality in the developed world, but vaccine efficacy, safety, and cost still pose a significant challenge to developing countries. Considering that the attack rate and mortality are relatively higher in developing countries, the control of rotavirus-attributable gastroenteritis mainly relies on vaccine coverage along with good hygienic measures. The introduction and expansion of the use of next-generation RV vaccines with better efficacy, safety, and low cost are necessary along with a multifaceted health approach to address the infections by rotavirus. A new generation of rotavirus vaccines will soon be licensed in many countries and available for more widespread use. Identifying the full value of these vaccines to prevent mortality from rotavirus in developing countries is still several years away and each of the vaccines must first show its effectiveness in poor populations in Africa and Asia. Although many hurdles remain to ascertain the effectiveness of these vaccines in key target populations and their affordability and to remove lingering concerns about safety from intussusception, the presence of two candidate vaccines provides an important new instrument to decrease the morbidity and mortality associated with rotavirus diarrhea.

DOI: http://dx.doi.org/10.5772/intechopen.109466

Author details

Kirti Nirmal* and Seema Gangar
Department of Microbiology, University College of Medical Sciences and Guru Teg Bahadur Hospital, Delhi, India

*Address all correspondence to: doctorkirtinirmal@gmail.com

References

[1] Bishop RF, Davidson GP, et al. Virus particles in epithelial cells of duodenal mucosa from children with viral gastroenteritis. Lancet. 1973;**1**:1281-1283

[2] Available from: https://www.who.int/westernpacific/health-topics/rotavirus-infections. [Accessed: October 4, 2022]

[3] Carstens EB. Ratification vote on taxonomic proposals to the International Committee on Taxonomy of Viruses (2009). Archives of Virology. 2010;**155**(1):133-146. DOI: 10.1007/s00705-009-0547-x

[4] Flewett T, Bryden A, Davies H, Woode G, Bridger J, Derrick J. Relation between viruses from acute gastroenteritis of children and newborn calves. The Lancet. 1974;**304**(7872):61-63. DOI: 10.1016/s0140-6736(74)91631-6

[5] Jayaram H, Estes M, Prasad BVV. Emerging themes in rotavirus cell entry, genome organization, transcription, and replication. Virus Research. 2004;**101**(1):67-81. DOI: 10.1016/j.virusres.2003.12.007

[6] Prasad BV, Burns JW, Marietta E, Estes MK, Chiu W. Localization of VP4 neutralization sites in rotavirus by three-dimensional cryo-electron microscopy. Nature. 1990;**343**:476-479

[7] Shaw AL, Rothnagel R, Chen D, Ramig RF, Chiu W, Prasad BV. Three-dimensional visualization of the rotavirus hemagglutinin structure. Cell. 1993;**74**:693-701

[8] Estes MK, Greenberg HB. Rotaviruses. In: Knipe DM, Howley PM, et al., editors. Fields Virology. 6th ed. Philadelphia, PA: Wolters Kluwer Health/Lippincott Williams & Wilkins; 2013. pp. 1347-1401

[9] Tihova M, Dryden KA, Bellamy AR, Greenberg HB, Yeager M. Localization of membrane permeabilization and receptor binding sites on the VP4 hemagglutinin of rotavirus: Implications for cell entry. Journal of Molecular Biology. 2001;**314**:985-992

[10] Settembre EC, Chen JZ, Dormitzer PR, Grigorieff N, Harrison SC. Atomic model of an infectious rotavirus particle. EMBO Journal. 2011;**30**(2):408-416. DOI: 10.1038/emboj.2010.322. Epub 2010 Dec 14

[11] Matthijnssens J, Ciarlet M, Heiman E, Arijs I, Delbeke T, McDonald SM, et al. Full genome-based classification of rotaviruses reveals a common origin between human Wa-Like and porcine rotavirus strains and human DS-1-like and bovine rotavirus strains. Journal of Virology. 2008;**82**(7):3204-3219. DOI: 10.1128/JVI.02257-07. Epub 2008 Jan 23

[12] Cohen J, Laporte J, Charpilienne A, Scherrer R. Activation of rotavirus RNA polymerase by calcium chelation. Archives of Virology. 1979;**60**(3-4):177-186

[13] Guo CT, Nakagomi O, Mochizuki M, Ishida H, Kiso M, Ohta Y, et al. Ganglioside GM(1a) on the cell surfaceis involved in the infection by human rotavirus KUN and MO strains. Journal of Biochemistry. 1999;**126**(October (4)):683-688

[14] Haselhorst T, Fleming FE, Dyason JC, Hartnell RD, Yu X, Holloway G, et al. Sialic acid dependence in rotavirus host cell invasion. Nature Chemical Biology. 2009;**5**(February (2)):91-93

[15] Coulson BS, Londrigan SL, Lee DJ. Rotavirus contains integrin ligand

sequences and a disintegrin-like domain that are implicated in virus entry into cells. Proceedings of the National Academy of Sciences of the United States of America. 1997;**94**(May (10)): 5389-5394

[16] Mackow ER, Barnett JW, Chan H, Greenberg HB. The rhesus rotavirus outer capsid protein VP4 functions as a hemagglutinin and is antigenically conserved when expressed by a baculovirus recombinant. Journal of Virology. 1989;**63**(April (4)):1661-1668

[17] Ludert JE, Michelangeli F, Gil F, Liprandi F, Esparza J. Penetration and uncoating of rotaviruses in cultured cells. Intervirology. 1987;**27**(2):95-101

[18] Periz J, Celma C, Jing B, Pinkney JN, Roy P, Kapanidis AN. Rotavirus mRNAS are released by transcript-specific channels in the double-layered viral capsid. Proceedings of the National Academy of Sciences of the United States of America. 2013;**110**(July (29)): 12042-12047

[19] Silvestri LS, Taraporewala ZF, Patton JT. Rotavirus replication: Plus-sense templates for double-stranded RNA synthesis are made in viroplasms. Journal of Virology. 2004;**78**(July (14)): 7763-7774

[20] Fabbretti E, Afrikanova I, Vascotto F, Burrone OR. Two non-structural rotavirus proteins, NSP2 and NSP5, form viroplasm-like structures in vivo. The Journal of General Virology. 1999;**80**(February (Pt 2)):333-339

[21] Berois M, Sapin C, Erk I, Poncet D, Cohen J. Rotavirus nonstructural protein NSP5 interacts with major core protein VP2. Journal of Virology. 2003;**77**(February (3)):1757-1763

[22] Taylor JA, O'Brien JA, Yeager M. The cytoplasmic tail of NSP4, the endo- plasmic reticulum-localized non-structural glycoprotein of rotavirus, contains distinct virus binding and coiled coil domains. The EMBO Journal. 1996;**15**(September (17)):4469-4476

[23] Crawford SE, Hyser JM, Utama B, Estes MK. Autophagy hijacked through viroporin-activated calcium/calmodulin-dependent kinase kinase-signaling is required for rotavirus replication. Proceedings of the National Academy of Sciences of the United States of America. 2012;**109**(December (50)):E3405-E3413

[24] Omatola CA, Olaniran AO. Rotaviruses: From pathogenesis to disease control—A critical review. Viruses. 2022;**14**:875. DOI: 10.3390/v14050875

[25] O'Ryan MG. Clinical Manifestations and Diagnosis of Rotavirus Infection: An Update. Wolters Kluwers. Available from: https://www.uptodate.com/contents/clinical-manifestations-and-diagnosis-of-rotavirus-infection#H3096970958. [Accessed: September 12, 2020]

[26] Bialowas S, Hagbom M, Nordgren J, Karlsson T, Sharma S, Magnusson KE, et al. Rotavirus and serotonin cross-talk in diarrhoea. PLoS One. 2016;**11**:e0159660

[27] Crawford SE, Ramani S, Tate JE, Parashar UD, Svensson L, Hagbom M, et al. Rotavirus infection. Nature Reviews Disease Primers. 2017;**3**:17083

[28] Lestari FB, Vongpunsawad S, Wanlapakorn N, Poovorawan Y. Rotavirus infection in children in Southeast Asia 2008-2018: Disease burden, genotype distribution, seasonality, and vaccination. Journal of Biomedical Science. 2020;**27**:66

[29] Yen C, Cortese MM. Rotaviruses. Principles and Practice of Pediatric

Infectious Diseases. Amsterdam, The Netherlands: Elsevier; 2018. pp. 1122-1125.e3

[30] World Health Organization (WHO). Rotavirus vaccines: An update. Weekly Epidemiological Record. 2009;**84**:533-537

[31] El Ageery MS, Ali R, NTA EK, Rakha SA, Zeid MS. Comparison of enzyme immunoassay, late x agglutination and polyacrylamide gel electrophoresis for diagnosis of rotavirus in children. Egyptian Journal of Basic and Applied Sciences. 2020;7:47-52

[32] Chen S, Wanga Y, Lia P, Yina Y, Bijveldsa MJ, de Jongea HR, et al. Drug screening identifies gemcitabine inhibiting rotavirus through alteration of pyrimidine nucleotide synthesis pathway. Antiviral Research. 2020;**180**:104823

[33] Center for Health Protection (CHP). Health Topics on Rotavirus Infection by the Department of Health, the Government of the Hong Kong Special Administrative Region. 2019. Available from: https://www.chp.gov.hk/en/healthtopics/content/24/38.html

[34] Soares Weiser K, Bergman H, Henschke N, Pitan F, Cunliffe N. Vaccines for preventing rotavirus diarrhoea: Vaccines in use. Cochrane Database of Systematic Reviews. 2019;**3**:CD008521

[35] Vesikari T, Matson DO, Dennehy P, Van Damme P, Santosham M, Rodriguez Z, et al. Safety and efficacy of a pentavalent human–bovine (WC3) reassortant rotavirus vaccine. The New England Journal of Medicine. 2006;**354**:23-33

[36] Vesikari T, Karvonen A, Prymula R, Schuster V, Tejedor JC, Cohen R, et al. Efficacy of human rotavirus vaccine against rotavirus gastroenteritis during the first 2 years of life in European infants: Randomised, double-blind controlled study. Lancet. 2007;**370**:1757-1763

[37] Bhandari N, Rongsen-Chandola T, Bavdekar A, John J, Antony K, Taneja S, et al. Efficacy of a monovalent human-bovine (116E) rotavirus vaccine in Indian children in the second year of life. Vaccine. 2014;**32**:A110-A116

[38] World Health Organization. Summary of Key Characteristics of Currently WHO-Pre-Qualified Rotavirus Vaccines, Version 1.4. 2019. Available from: https://www.who.int/publications/i/item/WHO-IVB-2021.03. [Accessed: November 10, 2022]

Chapter 3

Ocular Infection of HCMV: Immunology, Pathogenesis, and Interventions

Yan Yan and Renfang Chen

Abstract

Human cytomegalovirus (HCMV) retinitis accounts for 70% of herpesvirus-infected ocular diseases. Recent advances in knowledge of innate immune responses to viral infections have elucidated a complex network of the interplay between the invading virus, the target cells, and the host immune responses. Ocular cytomegalovirus latency exacerbates the development of choroidal neovascularization. Viruses have various strategies to evade or delay the cytokine response, and buy time to replicate in the host. Some signaling proteins impact the virologic, immunologic, and pathological processes of herpesvirus infection with particular emphasis on retinitis caused by HCMV. The accumulated data suggest that signaling proteins can differentially affect the severity of viral diseases in a highly cell-type-specific manner, reflecting the diversity and complexity of herpesvirus infection and the ocular compartment. By summarizing the immunological characteristics and pathogenesis of HCMV ocular infection, it will provide important information on the development of antiviral therapy, immunotherapy, and antidrug resistance.

Keywords: human cytomegalovirus (HCMV), retinitis, immunology, pathogenesis, resistance

1. Introduction

Human cytomegalovirus (HCMV) is a member of the beta-herpesvirus family, which tends to establish asymptomatic and lifelong latent infection [1]. Opportunistic HCMV reactivation is a common cause of increasing morbidity and mortality in newborns, the aged population, solid organ transplant patients, hematologic malignancy, or immunodeficient patients [2, 3].

HCMV was first reported to induce HCMV retinitis in 1957 [4], which is known to predominantly target retinal vascular endothelial cells, glial cells, and retinal pigment epithelial cells in the eye [5]. HCMV keratitis or retinitis is the most common opportunistic complication of infection in immunocompromised patients [2, 6, 7], including HIV-1-infected individuals. In general, HIV-1-infected individuals who have viral retinitis tend to be severe, long-lasting, and resistant to conventional treatment with a high rate of complications and significant visual morbidity [7].

Despite the widespread use of highly active antiretroviral therapy (HAART), up to 50–85% of AIDS patients develop ocular manifestations [8–10]. It has been well known that the HCMV can infect the immune-privileged retina site, lead to severe visual loss, and affect the quality of life in HIV-1-positive individuals [5]. Opportunistic infections develop when there is a deterioration of the immune status of the individual, which can be measured with the help of $CD4^+$ T-cell counts [5]. The proportion of HCMV retinitis manifestations was also correlated with the $CD4^+$ T-cell counts in patients [8]. Retinitis symptom has been classified into two categories, namely, infectious and noninfectious with the vast majority of manifestations occurring in the former. The infectious group mainly consists of the herpetic group of viral infections. Bacterial causes may be due to Staphylococcus epidermidis, Staphylococcus aureus, Pseudomonas aeruginosa, alpha-hemolytic Streptococcus, *Micrococcus*, and *Bacillus*. Fungal keratitis in HIV-1-infected individuals depend on the geographic locations from which the patient comes. *Microsporidia* and *Acanthamoeba* are common protozoal pathogens. Noninfective inflammatory causes include peripheral ulcerative keratitis, keratoconjunctivitis sicca, and squamous cell carcinoma of the conjunctiva. Posterior segment lesions caused by HCMV show severe visual disorders [7]. A severity that is abnormally severe or minimally reactive makes clinicians suspect immunosuppression. In the HAART era, the incidence, visual morbidity, and mortality of HCMV-related retinitis, and other HIV-1-related retinopathies showed a decline [8, 10]. In this chapter, we will focus on the immunological mechanisms and pathological processes of HCMV infection and strive to highlight those clinical manifestations that should alert the clinicians to suspect underlining HIV-1 infection and provide a basis for intervention.

2. Immunology of HCMV ocular diseases

2.1 Immunology

HCMV has evolved a variety of mechanisms to evade host immune surveillance and to establish latent infection with the ability to reactivate when the immune surveillance is compromised [11]. The host immune responses to HCMV involve both innate and adaptive immune systems, which play an important role in resolving both primaries, reactivating, and superinfections [12]. Under the innate and adaptive immune responses, a low viral load and latent state are established in the host after HCMV infection, but under the stimulation of the irregular and intermittent viral antigen reactivation, the functions of T-cells are exhausted [13]. At the same time, the HCMV virus can also encode a large number of gene products that interfere with the immune clearance responses to evade immune surveillance [11, 14, 15]. Considering that immunological clearance and evasion are associated with clinical outcomes, we summarized the immunological mechanisms of HCMV infection.

2.1.1 Innate immune responses

The natural killer (NK) cell is an important member of the innate lymphoid cell family for defense against HCMV during the early stages of infection and before the development of adaptive immune response due to its strong ability to kill infected or transformed cells [15]. The activities of NK-cells or NKT-cells (a subset of T-cells that co-express T- and NK-cell receptors) depend on the balance between activating and inhibitory signals transduced by its receptors [15]. They are also protected by releasing anti-viral cytokine interferon (IFN)-γ or by direct lysis, or autophagy of infected cells [15]. This will determine the disease progression of HCMV infection with ocular target cells.

2.1.2 Adaptive immune responses

Accumulating studies have shown that NK-cells take part in adaptive immune responses, such as clonal expansion and immune memory, during cytomegalovirus infection [16]. Clonal expansion not only serves to amplify the number of specific lymphocytes and mount robust protective responses against the pathogen but also results in the selection and differentiation of the responding lymphocytes [16]. In both innate and adaptive lymphocytes, clonal expansion is a critical process for host defenses. It has been shown that antigen (Ag)-specific T-cell expansion was estimated up to 400,000-fold [17]. The intensity of the adaptive immune responses suppresses the acute inflammatory responses caused by HCMV, causing less ocular tissue damage and sequelae.

In primary HCMV infections, $CD4^+$ T-cells play a vital role in controlling symptomatic disease in healthy and immunocompromised patients. It is important to note that HCMV-infected cells can induce impairment of HCMV-specific effector $CD4^+$ T-cell responses [18]. A subpopulation of HCMV-specific $CD4^+$ T-cells has been shown to express Foxp3 and to perform functions similar to regulatory T-cells, such as the production of IL-10 [18, 19]. Latent infection is associated with secretory expression of CCL8, IL-10, and TGF-β [13, 18]. The presence of viral genes and viral IL-10 lead to down-regulate human leukocyte antigen (HLA) class II molecules and limit antigen presentation to $CD4^+$ T-cells in antiviral immunity [12, 18]. At the peak of HCMV infection, HCMV-specific $CD4^+$ T-cells are $CD45RA^+$ $CD45RO^+$ and express $CD27^+$, $CD28^+$, $CD38^+$, and $CD40L^+$. During the latent infection period, the HCMV-specific $CD4^+$ T-cells are rich in $CD27^-$ $CD28^-$ $CD4^+$ T-cells (5–10%) [13]. It has been known that HCMV-specific $CD4^+$ T-cells are required for the maintenance of HCMV-specific $CD8^+$ T- and B-cell responses in adoptive T-cell immunotherapy in transplant patients [13]. $CD8^+$ T-cells undergo extensive expansion before differentiating into cytotoxic T-cells capable of producing high levels of cytokines, including IL-2, IFN-γ, TNF-α, perforin, and granzyme B [13]. For therapeutics, $CD8^+$ T-cells with long-term survival rates and the potential to respond to challenges are very useful in adoptive transfer strategies for treating HCMV infection. Therefore, HCMV-specific $CD8^+$ T-cell responses, including the maintenance, distribution, effector function, and metabolic requirements of these cells, have been highly interesting from a vaccine perspective.

Activated HCMV is typically controlled by $CD4^+$ and $CD8^+$ T-cell responses, while the virus replicates under the immunosuppressive condition and spreads rapidly to nearby tissues, resulting in worsening of retinitis, such as the patients accompanied with HIV-1 infection and chemotherapy for cancers. In addition to eliminating or perturbing surface immune recognition molecules (HLA I or HLA II molecules) from the antigen-presenting cells (B lymphocytes, dendritic cells, monocytes, or macrophages), HCMV immune evasion mechanisms have evolved to escape recognition and immune clearance of infected cells by effector cells through innate immunity, mimicked the inhibitory ligands or downregulate the activating ligands of NK-cells [11].

2.2 Pathogenesis of HCMV ocular diseases

Although HCMV infection can occur in healthy individuals, it is uncommon to observe symptomatic infection in individuals without immune suppression [3, 20]. HCMV retinitis is a clinical syndrome characterized by full-thickness necrotizing retinitis, which can result in profound vision loss, retinal detachment, and permanent vision loss [21]. The possible transmission paths of HCMV include blood, prenatal intrauterine infection, perinatal infection through breast milk or genital secretions, saliva, and sperm [22, 23].

In immunocompromised patients, primary HCMV infection causes severe complications, including pyrexia, viremic-septicemia, pneumonitis, and immunosuppression [24, 25]. In total, 60% of patients have been infected with HCMV prior to the onset of critical illness, and are commonly infected before adulthood [26]. It has been shown that patients who suffered HCMV reactivation during critical illness have ~2-flod the mortality rate of those who have not reactivated [27]. The clinical data suggest that the clinical outcome is not only the cause of HCMV replication but also the degree of virus-associated immune responses [3, 25]. In addition to HCMV and HIV-1 co-infected patients with lower $CD4^+$ T-cell counts have a higher risk of mortality, HCMV has sophisticated strategies to circumvent immunocyte recognition, such as changing the signals of immunomodulatory molecules and subverting T-cell and NK-cell function, and allowing it to establish lifelong infection in blood and bone marrow [16]. In these disorders, HCMV-infected individuals could be accompanied by hemophagocytic lymphohistiocytosis-associated genetic defects. The active and latent infection induce sustained systemic inflammatory responses and predisposes patients to produce autoantibodies, which increased the autoimmune disease progression [28]. It has been demonstrated that individuals infected with one HCMV strain may not necessarily be able to resist other HCMV strains [29]. HCMV also causes immunosuppression associated with T-cell exhaustion, which contributes to the persistence of infection [13].

HCMV retinitis is caused by lytic infection, the conclusion supported by clinical resolution with antiviral therapy. Healing is through fibrosis, which predisposes patients to future retinal detachment and is also the cause of severe vision loss [30]. When antiretroviral therapy is introduced, some individuals with HIV-1 develop immune-restorative uveitis, which is an inflammatory response to the presence of HCMV antigens in the eye by activating viral immediate-early gent product-2 and increasing FasL secretion [31]. This condition may cause more visual impairment in patients than potential retinitis [30]. One possible explanation is that the damage of HIV-1 infection to the blood-retinal barrier may contribute to the preferential entry of HCMV into the oculus [30].

2.3 Interventions of HCMV ocular diseases

Acute retinal necrosis was first described in Japan as acute unilateral panuveitis, retinal periarteritis, and necrotizing retinitis progressing to retinal detachment [32]. The symptoms of acute retinal necrosis include redness, ocular pain, photophobia, floaters, and blurred vision [32]. These studies suggest that the challenges in diagnosis and therapeutic challenges primarily in the absence of guidelines or evidence-based literature to follow [21].

Ganciclovir was licensed in 1989 and remains the only licensed drug sufficient to treat active HCMV infection. Although the oral prodrug valganciclovir was licensed in 2001, it delivers the same active ingredient. Ganciclovir-resistant HCMV disease has become a serious clinical problem in transplanted populations. Mutations in viral kinase (UL97) or polymerase (UL54) have been shown to mediate resistance to ganciclovir and valganciclovir [33]. For strains of HCMV-resistant to ganciclovir, foscarnet is used off-label. Thus, this field would benefit from more licensed drugs that are both safe and effective anti-HCMV [30]. This becomes particularly important for clinical trials seeking to test the anti-HCMV activity of novel compounds.

In large randomized controlled trials of HIV-1-associated HCMV retinitis in the era before combination anti-HIV treatment, in which the primary endpoint was an objective progression of CMV retinitis, an intra-ocular ganciclovir implant (15% of patients progressed after 100 days of treatment) was superior to intravenous ganciclovir (65% of patients progressed). The limitation of the intra-ocular ganciclovir implant was its failure to prevent CMV disease in the contralateral eye. In a subsequent randomized controlled trial of HIV-associated CMV retinitis, treatment with oral valganciclovir (38% of patients progressed after 100 days of treatment) was similarly effective to initial intravenous ganciclovir for 4 weeks followed by oral valganciclovir (45% of patients progressed). During the latter trial, most patients were also taking a combination anti-HIV treatment. As the ocular penetration of systemically administered anti-CMV drugs is limited, current clinical guidelines include consideration of intraocular injection of anti-HCMV drugs for patients who have sight-threatening HCMV retinitis

Agent	Route	Dosage	Side effects	Monitoring
Ganciclovir	IV	5 mg/kg 12 h for 2 wk	Myelosuppression, renal impairment, hepatic impairment, gastrointestinal symptoms, CNS disturbances; less well-tolerated	FBC, UEC, LFT
Valganciclovir	PO	900 mg BD for 3 wk		FBC, UEC, LFT
Foscarnet	IV	60 mg/kg 8 h for 2–3 wk; 90 mg/kg 12 h for 2–3 wk	Nephrotoxicity, hypocalcemia, hypomagnesemia (can lead to seizures), anemia, genital ulceration	FBC, UEC, calcium, and magnesium level
Cidofovir	IV	5 mg/kg once weekly for 2 wk; probenecid pre- and post-infusion	Renal impairment, neutropenia, ocular hypotony, iritis	FBC, UEC
Ganciclovir	Intravitreal	2–4 mg/0.05–0.1 mL	—	—
Foscarnet	Intravitreal	2.4 mg/0.1 mL	—	—
Cidofovir	Intravitreal	0.02 mg/0.1 mL	Narrow therapeutic window, retinotoxic	—

Abbreviations: IV, intravenous; PO, oral; BD, twice daily; FBC, full blood count; UEC, urea electrolytes creatinine; LFT, liver function test

Table 1.
Antiviral treatment for HCMV retinitis [32].

Agent	Bilaterality	Outcomes
Rituximab	Unilateral or bilaterality	Resolved
Basiliximab	—	Not reported
Anti-thymocyte globulin	Unilateral or bilaterality	Resolved
Alemtuzumab	Unilateral or bilaterality	Resolved and marked improvement
Natalizumab	Unilateral or bilaterality	Retinal detachment or blind
Ruxolitinib	Unilateral	Not reported
Tofacitinib	Bilaterality	Not reported

Table 2.
Biologic immunosuppression and HCMV retinitis [32].

(**Tables 1** and **2**). In addition to ganciclovir, given that the retina shows acute necrosis of one eye, corticosteroid or methylprednisolone is very important because of its effects in relieving intense inflammatory responses [21].

The HCMV persistent or progressive retinitis may be resolved by systemic administration of virus-specific cytotoxic T-cells (CTLs) [34]. HCMV-specific CTL therapy may become a novel monotherapy or adjunctive therapy, or both, for retinitis, especially in eyes that are resistant, refractory, or intolerant of antiviral therapies [34]. In addition, it has been demonstrated that HCMV strain-specific antibodies play an important role in preventing viral recrudescence after transplantation [29]. Antibodies, natural killer cells, and macrophages theoretically contribute to protective immune responses and are expected to interact and cooperate with T-cells to control HCMV replication. It was also recommended that studies of active immunization should proceed concurrently with passive immunotherapy using monoclonal antibodies with defined reactivity against specific proteins of HCMV against the resistance [34]. Recently, letermovir has been used in ganciclovir-resistant patients at doses of 720–960 mg, while intravitreal therapy with formic acid or ganciclovir was also used, and by monitoring continuous hematologic, renal, and hepatic function, some patients experienced an improvement in symptoms [32].

3. Conclusions

The interaction between HCMV and the host immune system is complex. NK-cells play an important role in the virus infecting the ocular target cells and take part in the processes of innate immune response and adaptive immune response. After the acute infection in adolescent accompanied by acute symptoms, the virus easily establishes latent infection and reactivate in immunodeficient HIV-1-infected and transplanted individuals. T-cell function is important in controlling HCMV recurrence. Immunodeficient individuals are susceptible to developing HCMV retinitis, which can be treated with systemic and intraocular topical medications, but are also prone to developing drug resistance. Therefore, understanding the immunology and pathogenic mechanisms of HCMV will help us further develop effective antiviral drugs for the treatment or mitigation of HCMV ocular disease.

Acknowledgements

This work was supported by the Wuxi Key Medical Talents Program (ZDRC024) and the Top Talent Support Program for Young and Middle-Aged People of the Wuxi Health Committee (BJ2020094).

Conflict of interest

The authors declare no conflict of interest.

Author details

Yan Yan[1,2] and Renfang Chen[2,3*]

1 Laboratory for Infection and Immunity, The Fifth People's Hospital of Wuxi, Affiliated Hospital of Jiangnan University, Wuxi, China

2 Hepatology Institute of Wuxi, The Fifth People's Hospital of Wuxi, Affiliated Hospital of Jiangnan University, Wuxi, China

3 Department of Infectious Diseases, The Fifth People's Hospital of Wuxi, Affiliated to Jiangnan University, Wuxi, China

*Address all correspondence to: 1094825330@qq.com

References

[1] Stern L, Withers B, Avdic S, Gottlieb D, Abendroth A, Blyth E, et al. Human cytomegalovirus latency and reactivation in allogeneic hematopoietic stem cell transplant recipients. Frontiers in Microbiology. 2019;**10**:1186. DOI: 10.3389/fmicb.2019.01186

[2] Zhang Y, Liang Y, Zhang X, Wang S, Cao J, Gao Z, et al. Pre-transplant platelet refractoriness and alternative donors are associated with cytomegalovirus retinitis in hematopoietic stem cell transplantation for severe aplastic anemia. Frontiers in Cellular and Infection Microbiology. 2022;**12**:870296. DOI: 10.3389/fcimb.2022.870296

[3] Munro M, Yadavalli T, Fonteh C, Arfeen S, Lobo-Chan AM. Cytomegalovirus retinitis in HIV and non-HIV individuals. Microorganisms. 2019;**8**:55. DOI: 10.3390/microorganisms8010055

[4] Allen A, Beeman HW, Christensen L. Cytomegalic inclusion disease. AMA Archives of Ophthalmology. 1957;**57**:90-99. DOI: 10.1001/archopht.1957.00930050098018

[5] Vogel JU, Fleckenstein C, Wagner M, Gumbel HO, Theegarten D, Cinatl J Jr, et al. The human eye (retina): A site of persistent HCMV infection? Graefe's Archive for Clinical and Experimental Ophthalmology. 2005;**243**:671-676. DOI: 10.1007/s00417-004-0965-0

[6] Radhakrishnan NSD, Venkatesh Prajna N, Rathinam SR. Corneal involvement in HIV infected individuals. Ocular Immunology and Inflammation. 2021;**7**:1-6. DOI: 10.1080/09273948.2021.1887283

[7] Banker AS, Chauhan R, Banker DA. HIV and opportunistic eye diseases. Expert Review Ophthalmology. 2009;**4**:173-185. DOI: 10.1586/eop.09.10

[8] Amsalu A, Desta K, Nigussie D, Delelegne D. Ocular manifestation and their associated factors among HIV/AIDS patients receiving highly active antiretroviral therapy in Southern Ethiopia. International Journal of Ophthalmology. 2017;**10**:776-781

[9] Sudharshan S, Kaleemunnisha S, Banu AA, Shrikrishna S, George EA, Babu BR, et al. Ocular lesions in 1,000 consecutive HIV-positive patients in India a long-term study. Journal of Ophthalmic Inflammation and Infection. 2013;**3**:2. DOI: 10.1186/1869-5760-3-2

[10] Luo J, Jing D, Kozak I, Huiming Z, Siying C, Yezhen Y, et al. Prevalence of ocular manifestations of HIV/AIDS in the highly active antiretroviral therapy (HAART) era: A different spectrum in Central South China. Ophthalmic Epidemiology. 2013;**20**:170-175. DOI: 10.3109/09286586.2013.789530

[11] Lucin P, Mahmutefendic H, Blagojevic Zagorac G, Ilic TM. Cytomegalovirus immune evasion by perturbation of endosomal trafficking. Cellular & Molecular Immunology. 2015;**12**:154-169. DOI: 10.1038/cmi.2014.85

[12] Lim EY, Jackson SE, Wills MR. The CD4+ T cell response to human cytomegalovirus in healthy and immunocompromised people. Frontiers in Cellular and Infection Microbiology. 2020;**10**:202. DOI: 10.3389/fcimb.2020.00202

[13] Vieira Braga FA, Hertoghs KM, van Lier RA, van Gisbergen KP. Molecular characterization of HCMV-specific

immune responses: Parallels between CD8(+) T cells, CD4(+) T cells, and NK cells. European Journal of Immunology. 2015;**45**:2433-2445. DOI: 10.1002/eji.201545495

[14] Fink A, Mikulicic S, Blaum F, Reddehase MJ, Florin L, Lemmermann NAW. Function of the cargo sorting dileucine motif in a cytomegalovirus immune evasion protein. Medical Microbiology and Immunology. 2019;**208**:531-542. DOI: 10.1007/s00430-019-00604-x

[15] Gao F, Zhou Z, Lin Y, Shu G, Yin G, Zhang T. Biology and clinical relevance of HCMV-associated adaptive NK cells. Frontiers in Immunology. 2022;**13**:830396. DOI: 10.3389/fimmu.2022.830396

[16] Adams NM, Grassmann S, Sun JC. Clonal expansion of innate and adaptive lymphocytes. Nature Reviews. Immunology. 2020;**20**:694-707. DOI: 10.1038/s41577-020-0307-4

[17] Badovinac VP, Haring JS, Harty JT. Initial T cell receptor transgenic cell precursor frequency dictates critical aspects of the CD8(+) T cell response to infection. Immunity. 2007;**26**:827-841. DOI: 10.1016/j.immuni.2007.04.013

[18] Mason MG, Poole E, Sissons JGP, Wills RM, John SH. Human cytomegalovirus latency alters the cellular secretome, inducing cluster of differentiation (CD)4+ T-cell migration and suppression of effector function. Proceedings of the National Academy of Sciences of the United Sates of America. 2012;**109**:14538-14543. DOI: 10.1073/pnas.1204836109

[19] Mason GM, Jackson S, Okecha G, Poole E, Sissons JG, Sinclair J, et al. Human cytomegalovirus latency-associated proteins elicit immune-suppressive IL-10 producing CD4(+) T cells. PLoS Pathoghology. 2013;**9**:e1003635. DOI: 10.1371/journal.ppat.1003635

[20] Doshi B, Khatib NZ, Phatak S, Modi R, Tiwari S, Subramanyam A. Do we need separate screening strategies for cytomegalovirus retinitis in different underlying immunosuppressed states? A retrospective study from Western India. Indian Journal of Ophthalmology. 2021;**69**:623-628. DOI: 10.4103/ijo.IJO_1398_20

[21] Dong X, Wee C, Xu D, Wan P. Rare cause of left eye floaters and blurred vision in an immunocompromised patient: Acute retinal necrosis (ARN). BMJ Case Reports. 2022;**15**:e248636. DOI: 10.1136/bcr-2021248636

[22] Cadena-Mota S, Munoz-Escalante JC, Martinez-Rodriguez LE, Bernal-Silva S, Tello-Martinez N, de la Torre-Rodriguez I, et al. Incidence of congenital and postnatal cytomegalovirus infection during the first year of life in Mexican preterm infants. Journal of Medical Virology. 2022;**94**:3349-3358. DOI: 10.1002/jmv.27705

[23] Xia W, Yan H, Zhang Y, Wang C, Gao W, Lv C, et al. Congenital human cytomegalovirus infection inducing sensorineural hearing loss. Frontiers in Microbiology. 2021;**12**:649690. DOI: 10.3389/fmicb.2021.649690

[24] Mansfield S, Griessl M, Gutknecht M, Cook CH. Sepsis and cytomegalovirus: Foes or conspirators? Medical Microbiology and Immunology. 2015;**204**:431-437. DOI: 10.1007/s00430-015-0407-0

[25] David A, Zeng D, Stewart P, Glomb N, Alcorn T, Jones S, et al. Cytomegalovirus viremia, mortality, and end-organ disease among patients with

AIDS receiving potent antiretroviral therapies. Journal of Acquired Immune Deficiency Syndromes. 1999;**38**:538-544

[26] Guidry CA, Mansfield SA, Sawyer RG, Cook CH. Resistant pathogens, fungi, and viruses. The Surgical clinics of North America. 2014;**94**:1195-1218. DOI: 10.1016/j.suc.2014.08.010

[27] Kalil AC, Florescu DF. Prevalence and mortality associated with cytomegalovirus infection in nonimmunosuppressed patients in the intensive care unit. Critical Care Medicine. 2009;**37**:2350-2358. DOI: 10.1097/CCM.0b013e3181a3aa43

[28] Gugliesi F, Pasquero S, Griffante G, Scutera S, Albano C, Pacheco SFC, et al. Human cytomegalovirus and autoimmune diseases: Where are we? Viruses. 2021;**13**:260. DOI: 10.3390/v13020260

[29] Martins PJ, Andoniou EC, Fleming P, Kuns DR, Schuster SI, Voigt V, et al. Strain-specific antibody therapy prevents cytomegalovirus reactivation after transplantation. Science. 2019;**363**:288-293. DOI: 10.1126/science.aat0066

[30] Griffiths P, Reeves M. Pathogenesis of human cytomegalovirus in the immunocompromised host. Nature Reviews. Microbiology. 2021;**19**:759-773. DOI: 10.1038/s41579-021-00582-z

[31] Chiou SH, Liu JH, Hsu WM, Chen SS, Chang SY, Juan LJ, et al. Up-regulation of Fas ligand expression by human cytomegalovirus immediate-early gene product 2 a novel mechanism in cytomegalovirus-induced apoptosis in human retina. Journal of Immunology. 2001;**167**:4098-4103

[32] Wu XN, Lightman S, Tomkins-Netzer O. Viral retinitis: Diagnosis and management in the era of biologic immunosuppression: A review. Clinical & Experimental Ophthalmology. 2019;**47**:381-395. DOI: 10.1111/ceo.13500

[33] Foulongne V, Turrière C, Diafouka F, Abraham B, Lastere S, Segondy M. Ganciclovir resistance mutations in UL97 and UL54 genes of Human cytomegalovirus isolates resistant to ganciclovir. Acta Virology. 2004;**48**:51-55

[34] Gupta MP, Koenig LR, Doubrovina E, Hasan A, Dahi PB, O'Reilly RJ, et al. Ocular outcomes after treatment of cytomegalovirus retinitis using adoptive immunotherapy with cytomegalovirus-specific cytotoxic T lymphocytes. Ophthalmol Retina. 2021;**5**:838-849. DOI: 10.1016/j.oret.2021.04.009

Chapter 4

Middle East Respiratory Syndrome Coronavirus Outbreaks

Abdulkarim F. Alhetheel and Faisal A. Alhetheel

Abstract

Middle East respiratory syndrome coronavirus (MERS-CoV) is a single-stranded RNA-enveloped virus that belongs to the Coronaviridae family. Initially reported in 2012 in Saudi Arabia, MERS-CoV is a zoonotic virus originating from bats and transmitted from camels to humans and among humans by contact. It causes both upper and lower respiratory tract infections and in some instances can lead to renal failure or death. This chapter provides an overview of the virologic aspects, outbreaks and risk factors, clinical symptoms, diagnostic methods, as well as prevention and management of MERS-CoV infection.

Keywords: MERS-CoV, outbreak, clinical symptoms, diagnosis, prevention

1. Introduction

The first case of the Middle East respiratory syndrome coronavirus (MERS-CoV) infection was reported in June 2012 in Saudi Arabia. MERS-CoV then spread to several neighboring countries, mainly Jordan and Qatar, and has since been reported in Asia, Africa, Europe, and America [1]. By October 16, 2018, 2260 confirmed cases and 803 deaths from MERS-CoV infection had been documented in 27 countries by the World Health Organization. The vast majority of cases (73%) were reported in Saudi Arabia, with only one widespread outbreak observed outside of the Arabian Peninsula in South Korea in 2015 [2]. Due to the high fatality rate (36%) [1], a lot of effort has been made to understand the origin and pathophysiology of this novel coronavirus strain to prevent it from becoming endemic in humans [3].

2. Middle East respiratory syndrome coronavirus

The first reported case of human MERS-CoV infection was in a 60-year-old man who was admitted to a private hospital in Jeddah, Saudi Arabia, on June 13, 2012. He presented with a 7-day history of fever, cough, expectoration, and dyspnea. He was a non-smoker, had no prior history of cardiopulmonary or renal disease, and was not maintained on any long-term medication. Vital sign examination showed a blood pressure of 140/80 mmHg, a pulse rate of 117 beats/minute, a temperature of 38.3°C, a respiration rate of 20 breaths/minute, and a body mass index of 35.1. Chest X-ray revealed low lung volume, bilateral enhanced pulmonary hilar vascular shadows more prominent on the left side, and accentuated bronchovascular lung markings. Multiple segmental, patchy, and veiling opacities were present in the middle and lower lung fields, and the costophrenic angles were mostly blunted. The cardiac silhouette was not enlarged, and the aorta was dilated and unfolded. Chest X-ray was repeated after 4 days, which showed that the opacities became denser and more confluent. Computed tomography performed 4 days after admission revealed few subcentimetric mediastinal and hilar lymph nodes, bilateral dependent airspace opacities with air bronchograms, scattered areas of ground-glass opacity, interstitial septal thickening, and nodularity in the upper lobes, with minimal bilateral pleural effusion. Collectively, these findings are suggestive of an infection. On the day of admission, oseltamivir, levofloxacin, piperacillin-tazobactam, and micafungin were started. Three days later, meropenem treatment was initiated, since meropenem-sensitive *Klebsiella pneumoniae* was identified in tracheal lavage sample collected on day 2. *Staphylococcus aureus* was detected in a sputum sample performed on admission. *Acinetobacter* was identified in tracheal aspirate collected on the day of death. No other pathogens were detected in respiratory specimens, and no bacterial growth was detected in blood samples.

The patient was transferred to the intensive care unit (ICU) for mechanical ventilation on the second day. Laboratory findings obtained on admission showed normal white blood cell counts except for a relatively high percentage of neutrophils (92.5%) and a low percentage of lymphocytes (4.3%). Liver enzymes, blood urea nitrogen, and creatinine levels were within the normal range. A small increase in the liver enzymes was noted from day 7 onward, with alanine aminotransferase levels of 20, 78, and 47 international unit (IU)/liter (l) on days 1, 7, and 8, respectively, and aspartate aminotransferase levels of 33 and 96 IU/l on days 1 and 8, respectively. The patient tested negative for the human immunodeficiency virus; however, testing for pneumocystis pneumonia was not performed. On the third day following admission, blood urea nitrogen and creatinine levels significantly elevated, and on the eighth day, white cell count began to rise and reached a peak of 23,800 cells per cubic millimeter by day 10, with neutrophilia, persistent lymphopenia, and progressive thrombocytopenia. Arterial oxygen saturation ranged from 78% to 98%. On day 11 (June 24, 2012), the patient died of progressive respiratory and renal failure [4].

2.1 The source of MERS infections

In 2012, a new coronavirus strain was detected in patients from the Arabian Peninsula with severe respiratory symptoms known as MERS-CoV. Camels were identified as the source of the infections; however, the role of these animals in transmitting the infection is not well understood. Approximately 300 isolated MERS-CoV genomes had been sequenced from humans and camels during the epidemic. Previous attempts to understand the MERS-CoV epidemic relied on these data or reports of case numbers; however, this led to conflicting results at odds with other sources of evidence. Nevertheless, Dudas et al. [5] determined the relationship among MERS-CoV strains and reconstructed their family tree by analyzing their sequenced genomes.

2.2 Genome structure and function

MERS-CoV, a lineage C betacoronavirus (BCoV), has a positive-sense single-stranded RNA (ssRNA) genome of approximately 30 kb (**Figure 1A** and **B**) [6, 7]. As of 2016, phylogenetic analysis of MERS-CoV had been performed on 182 full-length genomes and multiple concatenated genome fragments, including 94 from humans and 88 from dromedary camels [9, 10]. The MERS-CoV genomes share more than 99% sequence identity, indicating low mutation and variance rates. The MERS-CoV genome is divided into two clades: clade A, which contains only a few strains, and clade B, to which most strains belong [10].

Similar to other coronaviruses, approximately two-third of the 5′ end of the MERS-CoV genome consists of the replicase complexes open reading frame (ORF1a) and (ORF1b). The remaining one-third encodes the structural protein spike (S), envelope (E), membrane (M), and nucleocapsid (N) as well as five accessory non-replicating proteins (ORF3, ORF4a, ORF4b, ORF5, and ORF8b) likely involved in viral pathogenesis (**Figure 1B**) [6, 11–15]. Typical of coronaviruses, the MERS-CoV accessory proteins are not homologous with any known host or viral proteins other than those closely related to lineage C BCoV [10]. MERS-CoV structural and accessory protein-coding plasmids transiently transferred into cells showed that ORF4b is localized mostly in the nucleus, whereas all other proteins are localized in the cytoplasm (S, E, M, N, ORF3, ORF4a, and ORF5) [16]. In addition, MERS-CoV deletion mutations of ORFs 3–5 attenuate replication in human airway-derived (Calu-3) cells [17], while deletion mutations of ORFs 4a and 4b attenuate replication in hepatic carcinoma-derived (Huh-7) cells [14, 18]. This highlights the importance of MERS-CoV accessory proteins in viral replication *in vitro* [19].

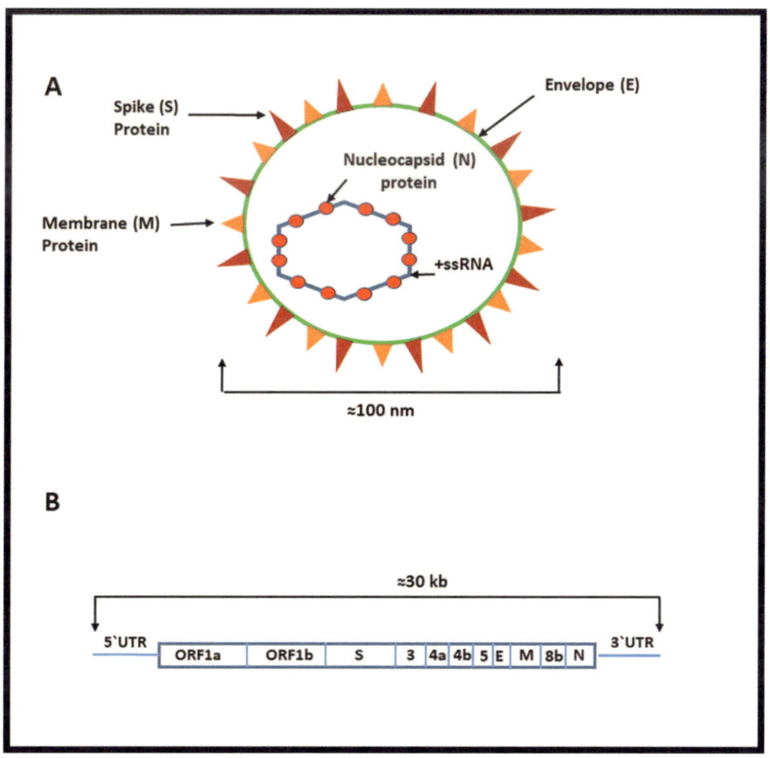

Figure 1.
MERS-CoV genome and schematic structure of viral proteins. (A) Schematic structure of major MERS-CoV structure proteins. (B) The MERS-CoV genome consists of two partially overlapping replicase open reading frames (ORF1a and 1b) and several ORFs that encode viral functional structural proteins and other proteins with unknown functions [8]. Abbreviation: MERS-CoV, Middle East respiratory syndrome coronavirus.

In response to viral infection, mammalian cells activate the type I interferon (IFN)-mediated innate immune response by producing type I IFNs (IFN-α and IFN-β). In contrast, evasion of host innate immunity through IFN antagonism, mediated by virus-encoded IFN antagonist proteins, is critical to viral pathogenesis. Each protein blocks key signaling proteins in the IFN and nuclear factor kappa B (NF-κB) pathways to enhance viral replication and pathogenesis [20–23]. Coronaviruses have evolved similar mechanisms to impede or bypass the innate immunity of their host at various levels, which ultimately contribute to viral virulence. Moreover, various coronavirus proteins disrupt signal transduction events required for the IFN response [24], often by interfering with host type I IFN induction.

MERS-CoV weakly induces type I IFN late during infection. In addition, MERS-CoV M, ORF4a, ORF4b, and ORF5 proteins are strong INF antagonists [16]. Studies using transient overexpression of the MERS-CoV accessory proteins ORF4a, ORFb, and ORF5 showed that they inhibit both IFN induction [16, 25, 26] and NF-κB signaling pathways [26]. MERS-CoV ORF4a, a double-stranded RNA (dsRNA) binding protein [25], potentially antagonizes antiviral IFN activity by inhibiting interferon production (IFN-beta promoter activity, IRF-3/7, and NF-kB activation) and the ISRE promoter element signaling pathway [16]. On the contrary, MERS-CoV ORF4b belongs to the 2H-phosphoestras (2H-PE) family and possesses phosphodiesterase (PDE) activity. Although MERS-CoV ORF4b is detected primarily in the nucleus of both infected and transfected cells [16, 25, 26], cytoplasmic expression levels are sufficient to inhibit activation of RNase L, a potent interferon-induced antiviral protein [16, 26]. MERS-CoV ORF4b was the first identified RNase L antagonist expressed by human or bat coronaviruses. It inhibits type I IFN NF-κB signaling pathways, providing a mechanism through which MERS-CoV can evade innate immunity [14, 26]. In addition, the MERS-CoV replicase nonstructural proteins (nsp1, nsp3, and nsp14) have been shown to interfere with innate immune signaling pathways through differing mechanisms [19, 27, 28]. In short, MERS-CoV has developed various mechanisms to evade the host immune system [29].

3. MERS-CoV infections and outbreaks

Between September 2014 and January 2015, a MERS-CoV outbreak resulting in 38 cases and 21 deaths was reported in Taif, Saudi Arabia. Clinical and public health records showed that 13 patients were healthcare personnel (HCP) and 15 patients, including 4 HCP, were associated with 1 dialysis unit. Serological studies done on three additional HCP in the same dialysis unit showed a positive report for MERS-CoV infection. Viral RNA was then measured from serum specimens of 15 patients in the acute phase, and full spike gene-coding sequencing was obtained from 10 patients, forming an unrelated cluster where sequences from 9 patients were closely related. Contrastingly, similar gene sequences among patients not linked by time or location suggest unidentified route of viral transmission. In short, circulation persists in multiple healthcare settings over an extended period, underscoring the importance of strengthening MERS-CoV surveillance and infection control practices [30].

Between May and July 2015, a large outbreak of MERS-CoV infection occurred in South Korea, which resulted from a traveler returning from the Middle East. This outbreak led to 186 confirmed cases in the country due to a primary case [31]. Patient 1 was diagnosed at Samsung Medical Center after transmitting the virus to several healthcare facilities. Patient 14 was exposed to Patient 1 outside the hospital and sought medical attention at the institution without knowing his infection status. Therefore, the experience gained from South Korea's first MERS-CoV case and a case following single-patient exposure in an emergency room showed the importance of investigating the epidemiology of MERS-CoV infection in a crowded areas such as an emergency room for the potential presence of super-spreaders [2].

4. MERS-CoV clinical features

MERS-CoV affects both upper and lower respiratory tracts in humans and may lead to complications ranging from renal failure to death. The symptoms in a patient with MERS-CoV are fever, sore throat, runny nose, and muscle ache. Some of the cases have developed to severe diseases by progression to acute respiratory distress syndrome. In severely ill patients, X-rays and other scans showed multilobar airspace disease [32].

Extra-pulmonary manifestations are common in severe cases; 30% of critical cases had gastrointestinal symptoms like nausea, vomiting, and diarrhea. Kidney disease has been reported for about 50% of critical MERS-CoV cases. Laboratory results showed leukopenia, lymphopenia, anima, and thrombocytopenia. Also, partial to moderate increase in amino transferase level is usual in MERS-CoV infection [32].

Herein we present the cases of two immunocompromised patients with MERS-CoV. In April 2013, two MERS-CoV cases were reported following nosocomial transmission from one patient to the other in a French hospital. Patient 1 visited Dubai, while patient 2 lived in France and had not traveled abroad. Both patients presented with fever, chills, and myalgia; however, patient 1 also complained of diarrhea. Respiratory status deteriorated, leading to acute respiratory failure requiring mechanical ventilation and extracorporeal membrane oxygenation (ECMO), and both patients experienced acute renal failure. MERS-CoV RNA was detected in lower tract specimens from both patients using reverse transcriptase polymerase chain reaction (RT-PCR) (e.g., cycle threshold [CT] values of 22.9 for upE and 24 for Orf1a from patient 1; CT values of 22.5 for upE and 23.9 for Orf1a from patient 2), whereas nasopharyngeal swab specimens were weakly positive or indeterminate. The patients shared a room for 3 days, and the incubation period was estimated to be 9–12 days for the second case. Patient 1 died on May 28 due to refractory multiple organ failure [33].

Another MERS-CoV case was presented in an old man with multiple myeloma. On March 8, a 73-year-old patient from Abu Dhabi developed flu-like symptoms with fever and a non-productive cough. He was admitted to the Mafraq Hospital in Abu Dhabi and was diagnosed with pneumonia. He was then intubated on day 9 due to progressive hypoxia and acute respiratory distress syndrome (fraction of inspired oxygen, 60%; positive end-expiratory pressure, 10 cm H_2O). The patient received intensive antimicrobial treatment with meropenem, levofloxacin, vancomycin, caspofungin, acyclovir, and oseltamivir during his stay in the ICU without major improvement of his pulmonary function. The patient was then transferred to the Klinikum Schwabing on March 19, 2013. Of note, relatives reported that the patients owned camels. He was diagnosed with multiple myeloma in 2008 and received several lines of treatment in the past few years, including high-dose chemotherapy with autologous stem cell transplantation in 2009. In November 2012, the patient had a relapse of multiple myeloma and was treated with lenalidomide and dexamethasone. During his stay in Munich, thrombocytopenia was observed. Interestingly, thrombocytopenia was also reported in early cases of MERS-CoV infection [4] including two of the four patients from a family cluster in Saudi Arabia [34] and two cases reported in France [33]. The patient then developed renal insufficiency on day 14 requiring dialysis. Despite continuous invasive ventilation and antibiotic treatment, the health status of the patient worsened, and he died on day 18 due to septic shock with signs of hemolysis and acute coagulation disorder [35].

On September 14, 2012, the United Kingdom Health Protection Agency (HPA) Imported Fever Service was notified of a case of unexplained severe respiratory illness in an ICU in London. The patient was a 49-year-old man who had recently been transferred from Qatar and had a travel history to Saudi Arabia. He developed mild undiagnosed respiratory illness while visiting Saudi Arabia in August 2012, which was fully resolved. On September 3, he presented to a physician in Qatar with cough, myalgia, and arthralgia and was prescribed oral antibiotics. Five days later, he was admitted to Qatar Hospital with a fever of 38.4°C and hypoxia (saturation of 91% in room air). Chest X-ray revealed bilateral lower-zone consolidation, and the patient required intubation and ventilation and was then transferred to London via air ambulance. The patient was clinically unstable and required manual ventilation during the transfer. On admission to the ICU in London, he remained severely hypoxic with arterial oxygen partial pressure of 6.5 kPA on 100% oxygen with optimized pressure ventilation. He required low-dose norepinephrine to maintain blood pressure. C-reactive protein was high (350 mg/L), and creatinine was high (353 μmol/L), with normal liver function and coagulation. The patient was treated with corticosteroids and broad-spectrum antibiotics, including meropenem, clarithromycin, and teicoplanin. Colistin and liposomal amphotericin B were later added. The patient's condition deteriorated with progressive hypoxia between September 11 and 20. His C-reactive protein level peaked at 440 mg/L and procalcitonin level at 68 ng/ml. His renal function also worsened, and hemofiltration was initiated on September 14. He was then transferred to a specialist ICU, and ECMO was initiated on September 20 (day 17 of illness). On October 2, he remained stable but was fully dependent on ECMO after 13 days (day 30 of illness) [36].

5. Diagnostic tests for MERS-CoV

MERS-CoV identification by diagnostic testing is crucial for tracking down cases of MERS-CoV, selecting appropriate treatment modalities to improve patient health, and lowering MERS-CoV symptoms and mortality rate. To date, RT-PCR is the mainstay test to diagnose MERS-CoV. However, like other tests, it has some limitations, including a long turnaround time and a lack of common measurements and correlations with viral load (VL). Most laboratories determine only CT values—which are inversely related to VL—to predict the viral concentration and disease progression as well as serve as a cut-off marker for diagnosis. However, few studies have evaluated the relationship between CT values and clinical severity [37]. Nevertheless, screening for MERS-CoV by RT-PCR upstream of the envelope gene (upE) is recommended, followed by confirming the presence of one of the following genes: open reading frame 1A, 1B genes, or nucleocapsid (N) [38]. Serology testing is another method to diagnose MERS-CoV.

Similar to other viruses, detecting antibodies and antigens by molecular methods may sometimes lag behind detecting the viral genome. To date, kinetics of antigen production in nasopharyngeal samples have not been studied. Moreover, viral antibodies usually appear 10 days after illness onset and are further delayed in severely ill patients requiring mechanical ventilation [39].

An enzyme-linked immunosorbent assay (ELISA) capture assay that can detect NP antigens of MERS-CoV virus in nasopharyngeal samples has been recently developed [40]. The assay is highly sensitive (detecting MERS-CoV-NP of less than 1 ng/mL) and specific (specificity of 100%) for MERS-CoV and can also be used in animals. Song et al. developed a rapid immunochromatographic assay to detect MERS-CoV nucleocapsid protein from camel nasal swabs, with a sensitivity of 93.9% and specificity of 100%. This assay is promising and worthy of replication in both camels and humans; however, antigen detection assays are not widely available. Nevertheless, this type of assay is valuable for ruling infections in or out.

Perera et al. [41] produced and optimized a microneutralization test to detect specific antibodies for MERS-CoV. Serial dilutions of serum sample were incubated with the Vero cells/MERS-CoV virus, and after 3-day incubation at 37°C, the antibody titers were scored based on virus cytopathic effect (CPE). Also, they developed a MERS-CoV spike pseudoparticle neutralization test [41], in which HIV/MERS spike pseudoparticles were used to infect Vero E6 cells. After 2 days, infected cells were lysed and antibodies that resulted in 90% luciferase reduction were reported as the ppNA antibody titer. As opposed to virus neutralization test, the pseudoparticle neutralization assay does not require biosafety level-3 (BSL3) containment.

An indirect immunofluorescent antibody assay to detect MERS-CoV antibodies was carried out using either whole virus in Vero cells [42, 43] or Vero cells transfected with MERS-CoV spike or nucleocapsid proteins [42]. ELISA utilizing S1 protein was also used to investigate the epidemiology of viral exposure [44]. To date, no studies have compared ELISA to either immunofluorescences assay (IFA) or neutralization assays.

Western blotting has been previously used to confirm antibody specificity to other viruses, such as SARS-CoV [45]. In addition, western blotting assays are needed to confirm antibody specificity in MERS-CoV, which can be in the form of genetically engineered specific MERS-CoV antigens blotted on the membrane.

Overall, MERS-CoV diagnostic testing and molecular techniques are the first-line methods used to confirm MERS-CoV infections. RT-PCR or sequencing of lower respiratory samples (tracheal aspirates and bronchoalveolar lavage samples) are recommended for viral detection. Thus, serological testing is a valuable tool to confirm suspected MERS-CoV cases; however, the virus cannot be detected in respiratory samples [46].

6. Prevention and treatment of MERS-CoV

Documenting the source of infection is key to preventing viral spread of MERS-CoV. Outbreaks are caused by viral transmission within healthcare settings facilitated by overcrowding, poor compliance with basic infection control measures, unrecognized infections, super-spreaders, and poor triage. However, actual contributing factors leading to MERS-CoV infection have not yet been systematically studied, but viral, host, and environmental factors are suggested to play major roles.

MERS vaccines can induce humoral and cellular immune responses. Specifically, a suitable MERS vaccine must induce a strong humoral immune response and, depending on the immunization route, activate B cells to produce systemic IgG and secretory IgA antibodies that bind to the virus and mediate systemic and mucosal responses [47–49], respectively. Serum IgA is also induced upon vaccination, particularly through the mucosal or intranasal routes [48]. The antibodies then neutralize MERS-CoV infection by blocking viral binding of the cell via the cellular receptor dipeptidyl-peptidase 4 (DPP4) and thus inhibiting cell entry [50, 51]. B cells can become antigen-specific memory B cells that can further boost immunization and induce rapid recall antibody responses [52]. However, this outcome has not been extensively studied in MERS-CoV vaccines.

Non-human primate (NHP) models were initially established as effective vehicles for MERS-CoV infection and vaccine evaluation; however, no vaccine against MERS-CoV is currently available for human use. Nevertheless, progress has been made since the emergence of the MERS-CoV in 2012. Unlike the SARS vaccines, which are developed based on attenuated or inactivated SARS-CoV and can potentially recover virulence factors [53–57], recombinant MERS-CoV vaccines can be developed based on recombinant viral particles using reverse genetics. For instance, a recombinant MERS-CoV with specific mutations is produced using a panel of contiguous cDNAs covering the whole viral genome and propagated to high titers in different tissue types. Additionally, an engineered mutant MERS-CoV that lacks the structural protein E was rescued and replicated in cells expressing the viral E protein [17, 18]. Using reverse genetics, developing replication-competent and propagation-defective MERS-CoV candidate vaccines that can provide a platform for designing live-attenuated MERS-CoV vaccines becomes possible. However, as recombinant MERS viruses contain major viral components and virulence factors, safety concerns need to be addressed, and their efficacy requires further assessment in appropriate animal models.

6.1 Viral-vector-based MERS vaccines

MERS vaccines can also be developed using viral vectors that express main MERS-CoV proteins, including the S proteins. As such, several MERS vaccine candidates have been produced and evaluated for immunogenicity in hDPP4-expressing mouse models and camels [47, 58–60].

Ad5 or Ad41 vectors expressing full-length S or S1 protein of MERS-CoV induce S-specific antibody and/or T-cell response in a mouse model via the intramuscular (IM) or intragastric route, effectively neutralizing MERS-CoV infection in vitro [58, 61]. In addition, IM or subcutaneous vaccination of mice with an MVA-based full-length S vaccine elicited the MERS-CoV challenge. Intranasally or intramuscularly administered MVA-S vaccine also induced mucosal immunity in camels, causing a significant decrease of excreted infectious viral RNA transcripts after MERS-CoV challenge. Similarly, a recombinant MV-based MERS vaccine expressing full-length or truncated S protein of MERS-CoV induced significant MERS-CoV, neutralizing antibodies and T-cell response, protecting mouse transducers with hDPP4 from the MERS-CoV challenge [62]. Although viral-vector-based vaccines can produce strong immune responses and/or protection, they may have unwanted safety and potency limitations.

6.2 Nanoparticle-based MERS vaccines

Nanoparticles can be used as delivery vehicles for MERS vaccines. The MERS-CoV full-length S protein can be prepared and purified from pellets of infected baculovirus insect cells. In the absence of adjuvants, nanoparticles induce a low level of MERS-CoV neutralizing antibodies in mice. However, by adding adjuvants such as aluminum hydroxide (Alum) or matrix M1, neutralizing antibodies become significantly increased and maintained. In addition, matrix M1 promotes increased production of neutralizing antibodies compared to alum [63]. Thus, adjuvants are required for MERS nanoparticle vaccines to promote immunogenicity. However, the efficacy and protection of this vaccine type have not yet been evaluated in MERS-CoV challenge models.

6.3 DNA prime/protein-boosted MERS vaccines

DNA priming followed by protein boosting could be used to develop MERS vaccines and subsequently expand DNA immunogenicity and efficacy. In this combined vaccination plan, DNA was constructed to encode the full-length MERS-CoV S protein, while the protein was expressed as the viral S1 subunit [64]. Studies have demonstrated that IM/electroporation priming of full-length S DNA and IM boosting of S1 protein of MERS-CoV with Ribi or alum (aluminum phosphate, AlPO4) adjuvant in mice and rhesus macaques induced robust neutralizing antibodies against MERS-CoV infection, conferring the protection of NHPs against MERS-CoV-induced radiographic pneumonia. However, the potential for vaccine-induced immune pathology needs to be investigated further.

6.4 Subunit MERS vaccines

Protein-based subunit vaccines against MERS-CoV have also been developed [49, 50, 65, 66]. While some subunit vaccines are designed based on the full-length S1 protein [64], most are based on viral RBD [49, 50, 65–67]. RBD-based vaccines have been evaluated for immunogenicity and protection in several MERS-CoV animal models, including hDPP4-transduced and hDPP4-Tg mice, as well as in NHPs [65–70]. The antigenicity and functionality of RBD proteins have also been extensively investigated.

Subunit vaccines do not induce the immune system as strongly as the other previously mentioned vaccines. However, the immunogenicity of subunit vaccines can be significantly enhanced by adding an ideal adjuvant via the appropriate route [48, 69]. In addition, maintaining a suitable conformation of the protein antigens in the vaccine, such as MERS-CoV RBD proteins [49, 50], is essential.

Subunit vaccines are the safest vaccine type since they do not contain viral genetic material. They are composed of antigens essential for developing protective immune responses, thus excluding the possibility of recovering virulence or inducing adverse reactions [71–73]. In contrast to vaccines based on the full-length S or S1 protein, RBD-based MERS subunit vaccines contain major neutralizing epitopes and lack non-neutralizing immunodominant domains; thus, they possess minimal risk of inducing non-neutralizing antibodies that can potentially lead to harmful immune responses or enhancement of virus infection [49, 74, 75]. This review aimed to provide guidelines for the development of effective and safe MERS vaccines.

7. Conclusion

With every passing years, our knowledge of MERS-CoV virus is improving; fewer cases of MERS-CoV have been reported as more studies improve our understanding of the virus. Appropriate diagnostic testing such as RT-PCR, documenting causes of viral outbreaks, and developing infection control units in every hospital have played key roles in hindering viral spread and preventing MERS-CoV from becoming endemic in humans, also lowering the risk of human infection by controlling animal-to-human transmission of the virus by vaccinating animals to prevent any transmission. There are studies that support developing potential therapies and vaccines to prevent infections [32].

Author details

Abdulkarim F. Alhetheel[1,2*] and Faisal A. Alhetheel[3]

1 Department of Laboratory Medicine, King Saud Medical City, Riyadh, Saudi Arabia

2 Department of Pathology, College of Medicine, King Saud University, Riyadh, Saudi Arabia

3 College of Pharmacy, King Saud University, Riyadh, Saudi Arabia

*Address all correspondence to: aalhetheel@ksu.edu.sa

References

[1] World Health Organization. WHO Statement on the third meeting of the IHR Emergency committee concerning Middle East respiratory syndrome coronavirus (MERS-CoV). Weekly Epidemiological Record. 2013;**88**(40):435-436. Epub 2013/10/29

[2] Cho SY, Kang JM, Ha YE, Park GE, Lee JY, Ko JH, et al. MERS-CoV outbreak following a single patient exposure in an emergency room in South Korea: an epidemiological outbreak study. Lancet. 2016;**388**(10048):994-1001. Epub 2016/07/13. DOI: 10.1016/S0140-6736(16)30623-7

[3] Bleibtreu A, Bertine M, Bertin C, Houhou-Fidouh N, Visseaux B. Focus on Middle East respiratory syndrome coronavirus (MERS-CoV). Médecine et Maladies Infectieuses. 2020;**50**(3):243-251. Epub 2019/11/16. DOI: 10.1016/j.medmal.2019.10.004

[4] Zaki AM, van Boheemen S, Bestebroer TM, Osterhaus AD, Fouchier RA. Isolation of a novel coronavirus from a man with pneumonia in Saudi Arabia. The New England Journal of Medicine. 2012;**367**(19):1814-1820. Epub 2012/10/19. DOI: 10.1056/NEJMoa1211721

[5] Dudas G, Carvalho LM, Rambaut A, Bedford T. MERS-CoV spillover at the camel-human interface. eLife. 2018;**7**. Epub 2018/01/18. DOI: 10.7554/eLife.31257

[6] van Boheemen S, de Graaf M, Lauber C, Bestebroer TM, Raj VS, Zaki AM, et al. Genomic characterization of a newly discovered coronavirus associated with acute respiratory distress syndrome in humans. MBio. 2012;**3**(6):1-9. Epub 2012/11/22. DOI: 10.1128/mBio.00473-12

[7] Wernery U, El Rasoul IH, Wong EY, Joseph M, Chen Y, Jose S, et al. A phylogenetically distinct Middle East respiratory syndrome coronavirus detected in a dromedary calf from a closed dairy herd in Dubai with rising seroprevalence with age. Emerging Microbes & Infections. 2015;**4**(12):e74. Epub 2015/12/04. DOI: 10.1038/emi.2015.74

[8] Song Z, Xu Y, Bao L, Zhang L, Yu P, Qu Y, et al. From SARS to MERS, Thrusting Coronaviruses into the Spotlight. Viruses. 2019;**11**(1):1-29. Epub 2019/01/17. DOI: 10.3390/v11010059

[9] Smits SL, Raj VS, Pas SD, Reusken CB, Mohran K, Farag EA, et al. Reliable typing of MERS-CoV variants with a small genome fragment. Journal of Clinical Virology. 2015;**64**:83-87. Epub 2015/03/03. DOI: 10.1016/j.jcv.2014.12.006

[10] Wernery U, Lau SK, Woo PC. Genomics and zoonotic infections: Middle East respiratory syndrome. Revue Scientifique et Technique. 2016;**35**(1):191-202. Epub 2016/05/25. DOI: 10.20506/rst.35.1.2427

[11] Lu R, Wang Y, Wang W, Nie K, Zhao Y, Su J, et al. Complete Genome Sequence of Middle East Respiratory Syndrome Coronavirus (MERS-CoV) from the First Imported MERS-CoV Case in China. Genome Announcements. 2015;**3**(4). Epub 2015/08/15.DOI: 10.1128/genomeA.00818-15

[12] Kim YJ, Cho YJ, Kim DW, Yang JS, Kim H, Park S, et al. Complete genome sequence of Middle East respiratory syndrome coronavirus KOR/KNIH/002_05_2015, isolated in South Korea. Genome Announcements.

2015;**3**(4):1-2. Epub 2015/08/15. DOI: 10.1128/genomeA.00787-15

[13] Kandeil A, Shehata MM, El Shesheny R, Gomaa MR, Ali MA, Kayali G. Complete genome sequence of Middle East respiratory syndrome coronavirus isolated from a dromedary camel in Egypt. Genome Announcements. 2016;**4**(2). Epub 2016/04/30. DOI: 10.1128/genomeA.00309-16

[14] Thornbrough JM, Jha BK, Yount B, Goldstein SA, Li Y, Elliott R, et al. Middle East respiratory syndrome coronavirus NS4b protein inhibits host RNase L activation. MBio. 2016;**7**(2):e00258. Epub 2016/03/31. DOI: 10.1128/mBio.00258-16

[15] Menachery VD, Mitchell HD, Cockrell AS, Gralinski LE, Yount BL Jr, Graham RL, et al. MERS-CoV Accessory ORFs Play Key Role for Infection and Pathogenesis. MBio. 2017;**8**(4). Epub 2017/08/24. DOI: 10.1128/mBio.00665-17

[16] Yang Y, Zhang L, Geng H, Deng Y, Huang B, Guo Y, et al. The structural and accessory proteins M, ORF 4a, ORF 4b, and ORF 5 of Middle East respiratory syndrome coronavirus (MERS-CoV) are potent interferon antagonists. Protein & Cell. 2013;**4**(12):951-961. Epub 2013/12/10. DOI: 10.1007/s13238-013-3096-8

[17] Scobey T, Yount BL, Sims AC, Donaldson EF, Agnihothram SS, Menachery VD, et al. Reverse genetics with a full-length infectious cDNA of the Middle East respiratory syndrome coronavirus. Proceedings of the National Academy of Sciences of the United States of America. 2013;**110**(40):16157-16162. Epub 2013/09/18. DOI: 10.1073/pnas.1311542110

[18] Almazan F, DeDiego ML, Sola I, ZunigaS,Nieto-TorresJL,Marquez-JuradoS, et al. Engineering a replication-competent, propagation-defective Middle East respiratory syndrome coronavirus as a vaccine candidate. mBio 2013;**4**(5):e00650-e00613. Epub 2013/09/12. DOI: 10.1128/mBio.00650-13

[19] Mielech AM, Kilianski A, Baez-Santos YM, Mesecar AD, Baker SC. MERS-CoV papain-like protease has deISGylating and deubiquitinating activities. Virology. 2014;**450-451**:64-70. Epub 2014/02/08. DOI: 10.1016/j.virol.2013.11.040

[20] Garcia-Sastre A, Biron CA. Type 1 interferons and the virus-host relationship: a lesson in detente. Science. 2006;**312**(5775):879-882. Epub 2006/05/13. DOI: 10.1126/science.1125676

[21] Garcia-Sastre A. Antiviral response in pandemic influenza viruses. Emerging Infectious Diseases. 2006;**12**(1):44-47. Epub 2006/02/24. DOI: 10.3201/eid1201.051186

[22] Randall RE, Goodbourn S. Interferons and viruses: an interplay between induction, signalling, antiviral responses and virus countermeasures. Journal of General Virology. 2008;**89**(Pt 1):1-47. Epub 2007/12/20. DOI: 10.1099/vir.0.83391-0

[23] Taylor KE, Mossman KL. Recent advances in understanding viral evasion of type I interferon. Immunology. 2013;**138**(3):190-197. Epub 2012/11/24. DOI: 10.1111/imm.12038

[24] Totura AL, Baric RS. SARS coronavirus pathogenesis: host innate immune responses and viral antagonism of interferon. Current Opinion in Virology. 2012;**2**(3):264-275. Epub 2012/05/11. DOI: 10.1016/j.coviro.2012.04.004

[25] Niemeyer D, Zillinger T, Muth D, Zielecki F, Horvath G, Suliman T, et al. Middle East respiratory syndrome coronavirus accessory protein 4a is a type I interferon antagonist. Journal of Virology. 2013;**87**(22):12489-12495. Epub 2013/09/13. DOI: 10.1128/JVI.01845-13

[26] Matthews KL, Coleman CM, van der Meer Y, Snijder EJ, Frieman MB. The ORF4b-encoded accessory proteins of Middle East respiratory syndrome coronavirus and two related bat coronaviruses localize to the nucleus and inhibit innate immune signalling. The Journal of General Virology. 2014;**95**(Pt 4):874-882. Epub 2014/01/21. DOI: 10.1099/vir.0.062059-0

[27] Lokugamage KG, Narayanan K, Nakagawa K, Terasaki K, Ramirez SI, Tseng CT, et al. Middle East respiratory syndrome coronavirus nsp1 inhibits host gene expression by selectively targeting mRNAs transcribed in the nucleus while sparing mRNAs of cytoplasmic origin. Journal of Virology. 2015;**89**(21):10970-10981. Epub 2015/08/28. DOI: 10.1128/JVI.01352-15

[28] Bailey-Elkin BA, Knaap RC, Johnson GG, Dalebout TJ, Ninaber DK, van Kasteren PB, et al. Crystal structure of the Middle East respiratory syndrome coronavirus (MERS-CoV) papain-like protease bound to ubiquitin facilitates targeted disruption of deubiquitinating activity to demonstrate its role in innate immune suppression. Journal of Biological Chemistry. 2014;**289**(50):34667-34682. Epub 2014/10/17. DOI: 10.1074/jbc.M114.609644

[29] Chafekar A, Fielding BC. MERS-CoV: understanding the latest human coronavirus threat. Viruses. 2018;**10**(2):1-22. Epub 2018/03/03. DOI: 10.3390/v10020093

[30] Assiri A, Abedi GR, Bin Saeed AA, Abdalla MA, al-Masry M, Choudhry AJ, et al. Multifacility outbreak of Middle East respiratory syndrome in Taif, Saudi Arabia. Emerging Infectious Diseases. 2016;**22**(1):32-40. Epub 2015/12/23. DOI: 10.3201/eid2201.151370

[31] Centers K, for Disease C, Prevention. Middle East Respiratory Syndrome Coronavirus Outbreak in the Republic of Korea, 2015. Osong Public Health and Research Perspectives. 2015;**6**(4):269-278. Epub 2015/10/17. DOI: 10.1016/j.phrp.2015.08.006

[32] Arabi YM, Balkhy HH, Hayden FG, Bouchama A, Luke T, Baillie JK, et al. Middle East Respiratory Syndrome. The New England Journal of Medicine. 2017;**376**(6):584-594. Epub 2017/02/09. DOI: 10.1056/NEJMsr1408795

[33] Guery B, Poissy J, el Mansouf L, Sejourne C, Ettahar N, Lemaire X, et al. Clinical features and viral diagnosis of two cases of infection with Middle East Respiratory Syndrome coronavirus: a report of nosocomial transmission. Lancet. 2013;**381**(9885):2265-2272. Epub 2013/06/04. DOI: 10.1016/S0140-6736(13)60982-4

[34] Memish ZA, Zumla AI, Al-Hakeem RF, Al-Rabeeah AA, Stephens GM. Family cluster of Middle East respiratory syndrome coronavirus infections. The New England Journal of Medicine. 2013;**368**(26):2487-2494. Epub 2013/05/31. DOI: 10.1056/NEJMoa1303729

[35] Drosten C, Seilmaier M, Corman VM, Hartmann W, Scheible G, Sack S, et al. Clinical features and virological analysis of a case of Middle East respiratory syndrome coronavirus infection. Lancet Infectious Diseases. 2013;**13**(9):745-751. Epub 2013/06/21. DOI: 10.1016/S1473-3099(13)70154-3

[36] Bermingham A, Chand MA, Brown CS, Aarons E, Tong C, Langrish C, et al. Severe respiratory illness caused by a novel coronavirus, in a patient transferred to the United Kingdom from the Middle East, September 2012. Euro Surveillance. 2012;**17**(40):20290. Epub 2012/10/20

[37] Feikin DR, Alraddadi B, Qutub M, Shabouni O, Curns A, Oboho IK, et al. Association of higher MERS-CoV virus load with severe disease and death, Saudi Arabia, 2014. Emerging Infectious Diseases. 2015;**21**(11):2029-2035. Epub 2015/10/22. DOI: 10.3201/eid2111.150764

[38] Shahkarami M, Yen C, Glaser C, Xia D, Watt J, Wadford DA. Laboratory testing for Middle East respiratory syndrome coronavirus, California, USA, 2013-2014. Emerging Infectious Diseases. 2015;**21**(9):1664-1666. Epub 2015/08/21. DOI: 10.3201/eid2109.150476

[39] Park WB, Perera RA, Choe PG, Lau EH, Choi SJ, Chun JY, et al. Kinetics of serologic responses to MERS coronavirus infection in humans, South Korea. Emerging Infectious Diseases. 2015;**21**(12):2186-2189. Epub 2015/11/20. DOI: 10.3201/eid2112.151421

[40] Chen Y, Chan KH, Kang Y, Chen H, Luk HK, Poon RW, et al. A sensitive and specific antigen detection assay for Middle East respiratory syndrome coronavirus. Emerg Microbes Infect. 2015;**4**(4):e26. Epub 2015/10/01. DOI: 10.1038/emi.2015.26

[41] Perera RA, Wang P, Gomaa MR, El-Shesheny R, Kandeil A, Bagato O, et al. Seroepidemiology for MERS coronavirus using microneutralisation and pseudoparticle virus neutralisation assays reveal a high prevalence of antibody in dromedary camels in Egypt, June 2013. Euro Surveillance. 2013;**18**(36):pii=20574. Epub 2013/10/02. DOI: 10.2807/1560-7917.es2013.18.36.20574

[42] Buchholz U, Muller MA, Nitsche A, Sanewski A, Wevering N, Bauer-Balci T, et al. Contact investigation of a case of human novel coronavirus infection treated in a German hospital, October-November 2012. Euro Surveillance. 2013;**18**(8):56-62. Epub 2013/03/02

[43] Corman VM, Muller MA, Costabel U, Timm J, Binger T, Meyer B, et al. Assays for laboratory confirmation of novel human coronavirus (hCoV-EMC) infections. Euro Surveillance. 2012;**17**(49):1-9. Epub 2012/12/13. DOI: 10.2807/ese.17.49.20334-en

[44] Muller MA, Meyer B, Corman VM, Al-Masri M, Turkestani A, Ritz D, et al. Presence of Middle East respiratory syndrome coronavirus antibodies in Saudi Arabia: a nationwide, cross-sectional, serological study. Lancet Infectious Diseases. 2015;**15**(6):629. Epub 2015/05/27. DOI: 10.1016/S1473-3099(15)00029-8

[45] Wang YD, Li Y, Xu GB, Dong XY, Yang XA, Feng ZR, et al. Detection of antibodies against SARS-CoV in serum from SARS-infected donors with ELISA and Western blot. Clinical Immunology. 2004;**113**(2):145-150. Epub 2004/09/29. DOI: 10.1016/j.clim.2004.07.003

[46] Al Johani S, Hajeer AH. MERS-CoV diagnosis: An update. Journal of Infection and Public Health. 2016;**9**(3):216-219. Epub 2016/04/24. DOI: 10.1016/j.jiph.2016.04.005

[47] Haagmans BL, van den Brand JM, Raj VS, Volz A, Wohlsein P, Smits SL, et al. An orthopoxvirus-based vaccine reduces virus excretion after MERS-CoV infection in dromedary camels. Science. 2016;**351**(6268):77-81. Epub 2015/12/19. DOI: 10.1126/science.aad1283

[48] Ma C, Li Y, Wang L, Zhao G, Tao X, Tseng CT, et al. Intranasal vaccination with recombinant receptor-binding domain of MERS-CoV spike protein induces much stronger local mucosal immune responses than subcutaneous immunization: Implication for designing novel mucosal MERS vaccines. Vaccine. 2014;**32**(18):2100-2108. Epub 2014/02/25. DOI: 10.1016/j.vaccine.2014.02.004

[49] Ma C, Wang L, Tao X, Zhang N, Yang Y, Tseng CK, et al. Searching for an ideal vaccine candidate among different MERS coronavirus receptor-binding fragments--the importance of immunofocusing in subunit vaccine design. Vaccine. 2014;**32**(46):6170-6176. Epub 2014/09/23. DOI: 10.1016/j.vaccine.2014.08.086

[50] Du L, Kou Z, Ma C, Tao X, Wang L, Zhao G, et al. A truncated receptor-binding domain of MERS-CoV spike protein potently inhibits MERS-CoV infection and induces strong neutralizing antibody responses: implication for developing therapeutics and vaccines. PLoS One. 2013;**8**(12):e81587. Epub 2013/12/11. DOI: 10.1371/journal.pone.0081587

[51] Zhang N, Tang J, Lu L, Jiang S, Du L. Receptor-binding domain-based subunit vaccines against MERS-CoV. Virus Research. 2015;**202**:151-159. Epub 2014/12/03. DOI: 10.1016/j.virusres.2014.11.013

[52] Ise W. Development and function of follicular helper T cells. Bioscience, Biotechnology, and Biochemistry. 2016;**80**(1):1-6. Epub 2015/06/30. DOI: 10.1080/09168451.2015.1056512

[53] Du L, He Y, Zhou Y, Liu S, Zheng BJ, Jiang S. The spike protein of SARS-CoV--a target for vaccine and therapeutic development. Nature Reviews. Microbiology. 2009;**7**(3):226-236. Epub 2009/02/10. DOI: 10.1038/nrmicro2090

[54] Tang L, Zhu Q, Qin E, Yu M, Ding Z, Shi H, et al. Inactivated SARS-CoV vaccine prepared from whole virus induces a high level of neutralizing antibodies in BALB/c mice. DNA and Cell Biology. 2004;**23**(6):391-394. Epub 2004/07/03. DOI: 10.1089/104454904323145272

[55] Takasuka N, Fujii H, Takahashi Y, Kasai M, Morikawa S, Itamura S, et al. A subcutaneously injected UV-inactivated SARS coronavirus vaccine elicits systemic humoral immunity in mice. International Immunology. 2004;**16**(10):1423-1430. Epub 2004/08/18. DOI: 10.1093/intimm/dxh143

[56] Zhou J, Wang W, Zhong Q, Hou W, Yang Z, Xiao SY, et al. Immunogenicity, safety, and protective efficacy of an inactivated SARS-associated coronavirus vaccine in rhesus monkeys. Vaccine. 2005;**23**(24):3202-3209. Epub 2005/04/20. DOI: 10.1016/j.vaccine.2004.11.075

[57] Jimenez-Guardeno JM, Regla-Nava JA, Nieto-Torres JL, DeDiego ML, Castano-Rodriguez C, Fernandez-Delgado R, et al. Identification of the mechanisms causing reversion to virulence in an attenuated SARS-CoV for the design of a genetically stable vaccine. PLoS Pathogens. 2015;**11**(10):e1005215. Epub 2015/10/30. DOI: 10.1371/journal.ppat.1005215

[58] Kim E, Okada K, Kenniston T, Raj VS, AlHajri MM, Farag EA, et al. Immunogenicity of an adenoviral-based Middle East respiratory syndrome coronavirus vaccine in BALB/c mice. Vaccine. 2014;**32**(45):5975-5982. Epub 2014/09/07. DOI: 10.1016/j.vaccine.2014.08.058

[59] Song F, Fux R, Provacia LB, Volz A, Eickmann M, Becker S, et al. Middle

East respiratory syndrome coronavirus spike protein delivered by modified vaccinia virus Ankara efficiently induces virus-neutralizing antibodies. Journal of Virology. 2013;**87**(21):11950-11954. Epub 2013/08/30. DOI: 10.1128/JVI.01672-13

[60] Volz A, Kupke A, Song F, Jany S, Fux R, Shams-Eldin H, et al. Protective efficacy of recombinant modified vaccinia virus Ankara delivering Middle East respiratory syndrome coronavirus spike glycoprotein. Journal of Virology. 2015;**89**(16):8651-8656. Epub 2015/05/29. DOI: 10.1128/JVI.00614-15

[61] Guo X, Deng Y, Chen H, Lan J, Wang W, Zou X, et al. Systemic and mucosal immunity in mice elicited by a single immunization with human adenovirus type 5 or 41 vector-based vaccines carrying the spike protein of Middle East respiratory syndrome coronavirus. Immunology. 2015;**145**(4):476-484. Epub 2015/03/13. DOI: 10.1111/imm.12462

[62] Malczyk AH, Kupke A, Prufer S, Scheuplein VA, Hutzler S, Kreuz D, et al. A highly immunogenic and protective Middle East respiratory syndrome coronavirus vaccine based on a recombinant Measles virus vaccine platform. Journal of Virology. 2015;**89**(22):11654-11667. Epub 2015/09/12. DOI: 10.1128/JVI.01815-15

[63] Coleman CM, Liu YV, Mu H, Taylor JK, Massare M, Flyer DC, et al. Purified coronavirus spike protein nanoparticles induce coronavirus neutralizing antibodies in mice. Vaccine. 2014;**32**(26):3169-3174. Epub 2014/04/17. DOI: 10.1016/j.vaccine.2014.04.016

[64] Wang L, Shi W, Joyce MG, Modjarrad K, Zhang Y, Leung K, et al. Evaluation of candidate vaccine approaches for MERS-CoV. Nature Communications. 2015;**6**:7712. Epub 2015/07/29. DOI: 10.1038/ncomms8712

[65] Lan J, Deng Y, Chen H, Lu G, Wang W, Guo X, et al. Tailoring subunit vaccine immunity with adjuvant combinations and delivery routes using the Middle East respiratory coronavirus (MERS-CoV) receptor-binding domain as an antigen. PLoS One. 2014;**9**(11):e112602. Epub 2014/11/19. DOI: 10.1371/journal.pone.0112602

[66] Lan J, Yao Y, Deng Y, Chen H, Lu G, Wang W, et al. Recombinant receptor binding domain protein induces partial protective immunity in Rhesus Macaques against Middle East respiratory syndrome coronavirus challenge. eBioMedicine. 2015;**2**(10):1438-1446. Epub 2015/12/03. DOI: 10.1016/j.ebiom.2015.08.031

[67] Mou H, Raj VS, van Kuppeveld FJ, Rottier PJ, Haagmans BL, Bosch BJ. The receptor binding domain of the new Middle East respiratory syndrome coronavirus maps to a 231-residue region in the spike protein that efficiently elicits neutralizing antibodies. Journal of Virology. 2013;**87**(16):9379-9383. Epub 2013/06/21. DOI: 10.1128/JVI.01277-13

[68] Tao X, Garron T, Agrawal AS, Algaissi A, Peng BH, Wakamiya M, et al. Characterization and demonstration of the value of a Lethal Mouse Model of Middle East respiratory syndrome coronavirus infection and disease. Journal of Virology. 2016;**90**(1):57-67. Epub 2015/10/09. DOI: 10.1128/JVI.02009-15

[69] Zhang N, Channappanavar R, Ma C, Wang L, Tang J, Garron T, et al. Identification of an ideal adjuvant for receptor-binding domain-based subunit vaccines against Middle East respiratory syndrome coronavirus. Cellular & Molecular Immunology. 2016;**13**(2):180-190. Epub 2015/02/03. DOI: 10.1038/cmi.2015.03

[70] Du L, Zhao G, Kou Z, Ma C, Sun S, Poon VK, et al. Identification of a

receptor-binding domain in the S protein of the novel human coronavirus Middle East respiratory syndrome coronavirus as an essential target for vaccine development. Journal of Virology. 2013;**87**(17):9939-9942. Epub 2013/07/05. DOI: 10.1128/JVI.01048-13

[71] Chlibek R, Pauksens K, Rombo L, van Rijckevorsel G, Richardus JH, Plassmann G, et al. Long-term immunogenicity and safety of an investigational herpes zoster subunit vaccine in older adults. Vaccine. 2016;**34**(6):863-868. Epub 2015/10/04. DOI: 10.1016/j.vaccine.2015.09.073

[72] Berkowitz EM, Moyle G, Stellbrink HJ, Schurmann D, Kegg S, Stoll M, et al. Safety and immunogenicity of an adjuvanted Herpes Zoster subunit candidate vaccine in HIV-infected adults: a phase 1/2a randomized, placebo-controlled study. Journal of Infectious Diseases. 2015;**211**(8):1279-1287. Epub 2014/11/06. DOI: 10.1093/infdis/jiu606

[73] Durando P, Fenoglio D, Boschini A, Ansaldi F, Icardi G, Sticchi L, et al. Safety and immunogenicity of two influenza virus subunit vaccines, with or without MF59 adjuvant, administered to human immunodeficiency virus type 1-seropositive and -seronegative adults. Clinical and Vaccine Immunology. 2008;**15**(2):253-259. Epub 2007/11/16. DOI: 10.1128/CVI.00316-07

[74] Zhang N, Jiang S, Du L. Current advancements and potential strategies in the development of MERS-CoV vaccines. Expert Review of Vaccines. 2014;**13**(6):761-774. Epub 2014/04/29. DOI: 10.1586/14760584.2014.912134

[75] Du L, Jiang S. Middle East respiratory syndrome: current status and future prospects for vaccine development. Expert Opinion on Biological Therapy. 2015;**15**(11):1647-1651. Epub 2015/09/29. DOI: 10.1517/14712598.2015.1092518

Chapter 5

A Review on Viral Outbreak in India with Special Reference to COVID-19

Aishwarya Khamari, Monika Khamari, Akshya Kumar Mishra, Jijnasa Panda, Debashish Gardia and Ratikanta Rath

Abstract

COVID-19, Middle East respiratory syndrome (MERS), and SARS are three severe pandemics linked to novel coronaviruses that have so far impacted people in the twenty first century. These acute respiratory tract infections (ARTIs) are brought on by viruses that are all exceedingly contagious and/or have caused large mortality. On January 7, 2020, a patient in Wuhan, China, with pneumonia-like symptoms had a novel coronavirus found in lung fluid. In 1980, the smallpox disease was formally deemed extinct worldwide. The cause of smallpox is unknown. The discovery of smallpox-like lesions on Egyptian mummies indicates that the illness has existed for at least 3000 years. The Ebola virus, a member of the filovirus family that affects both humans and other primates, causes the severe illness known as Ebola virus disease (EVD). The idea that swine influenza was a sickness related to human flu was originally put forth when pigs were ill during the 1918 flu pandemic at the same time as humans. Because viruses vary in their structural, anatomical, and molecular makeup, distinct viral diseases can be detected or tested using different methodologies, procedures, or diagnostic tools. Viral vaccines come in a wide variety of varieties in the pharmaceutical industry. From a medical perspective, several treatments are used for various viral illnesses.

Keywords: COVID-19, flu, testing, outbreak, treatment, Indian context, pandemics, Ebola virus disease

1. Introduction

COVID-19, Middle East respiratory syndrome (MERS), and SARS are three severe pandemics linked to novel coronaviruses that have so far impacted people in the twenty first century. These acute respiratory tract infections (ARTIs) are brought on by viruses that are all exceedingly contagious and/or have caused large mortality. Another zoonotic novel coronavirus with the name severe acute respiratory syndrome coronavirus 2 is the cause of the recently identified COVID-19 sickness, a highly contagious viral infection (SARS-CoV-2). Similar to the other two coronaviruses like SARS-CoV-1 and MERS-CoV, SARS-CoV-2 is most likely to have originated from bats, which have long served as established reservoirs for a range of lethal coronaviruses [1]. In December 2019, there were several reports of individuals in the province of Hubei who were admitted to hospitals with a brand-new illness characterised by pneumonia and respiratory failure and brought on by a novel coronavirus (SARS-CoV-2) (China). On February 11, 2020, the World Health Organization (WHO) identified this agent as the COVID-19 causal agent. 2019 (Coronavirus Disease). Despite the use of significant containment measures, the disease later spread to other Asian countries, the Middle East, and Europe. On March 11, Tedros Adhanom Ghebreyesus, the director general of the WHO, said that COVID-19 was a pandemic [2, 3].

Numerous studies show that after the coronavirus infection (COVID-19) outbreak, anxiety around it has significantly increased. To measure COVID-19 fear, a number of questionnaires have been developed concurrently. The several questions could cover a wide range of subjects, and COVID-19 dread is not necessarily a widely accepted idea. We conducted structural equation modelling and network analysis on four scales in an online convenience sample to examine the underlying structure of COVID-19 fear [4].

It is more crucial to comprehend the organisation and structure of conspiracy theories and misleading information about the COVID-19 epidemic in order to counteract the harm that these dubious claims pose as the pandemic spreads. We found distinct belief clusters when surveying Americans on their views on 11 of these ideas. These belief clusters correlated with various individual-level traits (like support for Trump and mistrust of scientists) and behavioural intentions (like taking a vaccine or participating in social activities) [5].

The rapid development of diagnostics for the novel virus was made possible by the genome assembly and release of the severe acute respiratory syndrome coronavirus 2 (SARS-CoV-2) in January 2020. Due to this, the largest global testing programme in history was launched and has since tested hundreds of millions of people. The massive amount of testing has stimulated innovation in the techniques, instruments, and theories that direct public health testing [6].

Physical isolation has been recommended as one of the most effective techniques to inhibit the transmission of COVID-19 before a vaccine or efficient therapy is created. How far people can be physically apart depending on both population density and behavioural characteristics. Most models developed to predict the spread of COVID-19 in the US do not explicitly take population density into account [7].

The Centres for Illness Control and Prevention developed and conducted the initial test as a result of the novel coronavirus severe acute respiratory syndrome coronavirus 2 producing coronavirus disease 2019 cases in the United States. The Centres for Disease Control and Prevention had to use the Emergency Utilization Authorization to allow both university and commercial labs to develop assays for determining the virus's existence as the number of cases increased and the necessity for testing increased. Several nucleic acid assays were developed on the basis of RT-PCR, each with its own techniques, specifications, and turnaround times. The pandemic-like spread of the illnesses made testing even more crucial. Prioritisation was required in accordance with instructions because the test supply ran out before it could satisfy demand [8].

Due to the breakdown of global cooperation and a lack of international solidarity, several low- and medium-income countries have been refused access to clinical tools in the COVID-19 pandemic response. Despite the availability and scalability of fast immunodiagnostic testing, knowledge of the dynamics of the immune response associated with infection is lacking [9].

The US has given ongoing emphasis to the value of testing in decreasing and suppressing the spread of the severe acute respiratory syndrome coronavirus 2 (SARS-CoV-2). Due to problems with test validation at the Centres for Illness Control and Prevention, testing was put off after the first case of coronavirus disease 2019 (COVID-19) was identified in the US in mid-January 2020 [10, 11].

The coronavirus disease (COVID-19) pandemic has shifted the focus of the global discussion about how to end the epidemic to the clinical lab and SARS-CoV-2 tests. Clinical laboratories have developed, approved, and used a variety of molecular and serologic assays to look for SARS-CoV-2 infection as a result. This has been essential for identifying cases, directing isolation decisions, and controlling the transmission of disease [12].

2. History

2.1 History of COVID-19

On January 7, 2020, a patient in Wuhan, China, with pneumonia-like symptoms had a novel coronavirus found in lung fluid. On January 10, 2020, the severe acute respiratory syndrome coronavirus 2 (SARS-CoV-2) assembled reference genome was revealed, and the first diagnostic tests to detect the virus were made available 2 weeks later. Since hundreds of millions of people have been tested for SARS-CoV-2, there has been a great deal of interest in and debate regarding diagnostic theories and procedures. In Wuhan, China, the first SARS-CoV-2 infections were found. It is still uncertain how the virus initially infected humans and if it turned into a pathogen before to or following the spillover incidence. The fifth known pandemic since the 1918 flu pandemic was caused by the uncommon human coronavirus disease of 2019 (COVID-19), which was originally discovered in Wuhan, China, in 2019. More than 200 million confirmed cases and more than 4.6 million fatalities had been reported as of September 2021, around 2°years after COVID-19 was first discovered. In this article, we present a thorough examination of the development of COVID-19, from the first case ever reported to the most recent efforts to stop the disease's global spread through vaccine campaigns. The World Health Organization (WHO) in Wuhan, China, received reports of pneumonia episodes on December 31, 2019, and as a result, the first COVID-19 cases were found. On January 7, the Chinese government determined that these instances were brought on by the 2019-nCoV, a brand-new coronavirus. A few weeks later, on January 30, 2020, the WHO deemed the fast expanding COVID-19 epidemic a Public Health Emergency of International Concern. The new coronavirus wasn't officially given a name until February 11th, when COVID-19 was assigned. The first instances of COVID-19 were discovered after reports of pneumonia episodes were received by the World Health Organization (WHO) in Wuhan, China, on December 31, 2019. The rapidly spreading COVID-19 epidemic was classified as a Public Health Emergency of International Concern by the WHO a few weeks later, on January 30, 2020. On February 11th, COVID-19 was given as the novel coronavirus's official name [1, 13–17].

2.2 History of smallpox

The cause of smallpox is unknown. The discovery of smallpox-like lesions on Egyptian mummies indicates that the illness has existed for at least 3000 years. The first written account of a disease akin to smallpox was produced in China during the fourth century CE (Common Era). India saw one of the worst smallpox epidemics of the twentieth century in 1974, 3 years before smallpox was completely eradicated. More than 15,000 people contracted smallpox and died as a result between January and May 1974. West Bengal, Bihar, and Odisha are three Indian states where the majority of the fatalities occurred. There were many thousands of people who were still alive but were either blind or deformed. India reported 61,482 smallpox cases to the World Health Organization (WHO) during these 5 months. In 1974, India was home to over 86% of all smallpox cases in the globe, primarily as a result of this pandemic. On May 24, 1975, a smallpox patient was found in India, and by January 1975, an operation known as "Target Zero" had been started in an effort to eradicate all remaining cases. In 1980, the smallpox disease was formally deemed extinct worldwide. Despite the fact that this programme was first introduced in 1958, it did not move swiftly because of disagreements between the WHO and the Indian government on logistics. Progress was only truly accomplished after the WHO was reorganised in the middle of the 1960s in India. Donald Henderson, a U.S. Public Health Services Officer in New Delhi, said that "If this attention and concern can last for the foreseeable future, smallpox will be eliminated. Everything seems to be in working order, though we don't think we're being overconfident. By June 1975, we hope to have eradicated smallpox in Asia" [18–23].

2.3 History of Ebola

History of the disease. The Ebola virus, a member of the filovirus family that affects both humans and other primates, causes the severe illness known as Ebola virus disease (EVD). The illness almost simultaneously spread to the Democratic Republic of the Congo (DRC) and Sudan in 1976 (now South Sudan). An EVD outbreak was reported in the Beni Health Zone in North Kivu Province on October 8, the DRC's Ministry of Health reported. Three suspected cases were later discovered in September 2021, and other cases in the same health zone were eventually confirmed. Sequencing results revealed a connection to the outbreak that struck the same area in 2018–2020, demonstrating that an EVD survivor's chronic infection was most likely the root cause of this outbreak. On December 16, 2021, 42 days after the final confirmed patient was removed from care, the 13th EVD outbreak in the DRC was ruled to be over legally. The Democratic Republic of the Congo's Ministry of Health (MOH) revealed on February 7, 2021 that an Ebola virus disease (EVD) case had been identified in North Kivu Province's Biena Health Zone. Later incidents were verified. EVD was present in North Kivu prior to the largest Ebola outbreak in the DRC's history, which occurred from 2018 to 2020 and was declared over on June 25, 2020. According to sample sequencing, cases from the 2018 to 2020 outbreak are connected to patients in this pandemic. It is likely that these cases resulted from sexual transmission of the virus or from a survivor who relapsed with a chronic infection. On May 3, 2021, the outbreak was determined to be over. On June 1, 2020, the DRC government announced a fresh Ebola outbreak in Mbandaka, Equateur Province of western DRC. The DRC government received technical support from international partners including the CDC to aid in response operations. This outbreak, the eleventh to hit the DRC, started as the tenth was still rapidly expanding over the east of the country. The DRC government announced the 10th Ebola epidemic on August 1 in the nation's eastern North Kivu province. Instances were also reported in the provinces of South Kivu and Uganda. In order to coordinate efforts and offer technical advice regarding laboratory testing, contact tracing, infection control, border health screening, data management, risk communication and health education, vaccination, and logistics, the CDC worked with the DRC government, neighbouring nations, local and international partners. A number of probable Ebola virus disease (EVD) cases were reported in the Likati health zone in the province of Bas Uele on May 11 by the Democratic Republic of the Congo's Ministry of Public Health, which also alerted other international public health organisations to the situation. Eight suspected instances, including two fatalities, were listed in the original report. On May 12, there was word of a third fatality. Two samples proved positive for Ebola Zaire during testing by the Institute National de Recherche Biomédicale (INRB) in Kinshasa. Health's epidemiologic, diagnostic, clinical, and communication efforts to contain the outbreak were supported by teams from international organisations like the CDC, WHO, MSF (Doctors without Borders), and others. The outbreak solely impacted the western province of Equator, even though it spread to several villages close to the town of Boende. The Ebola virus strain that caused it, meanwhile, was quite similar to the one that was responsible for the outbreak in Kikwit in 1995. This outbreak had nothing to do with the significant outbreak that was happening concurrently in West Africa. The probable death of an EVD patient was reported by the Uganda Ministry of Health on May 6, 2011. The Uganda Virus Research Institute's newly created CDC Viral Haemorrhagic Fever lab quickly identified the Ebola virus in a blood sample (UVRI). This outbreak was contained in part by the ability to quickly confirm the presence of the Ebola virus through laboratory testing carried out in-country, the clinical staff's early, strong suspicion of hemorrhagic fever, the appropriate use of personal protective equipment and barrier methods to safeguard hospital staff, and the ability to quickly stop the spread of the virus [24–28].

2.4 History of swine flu

The idea that swine influenza was a sickness related to human flu was originally put forth when pigs were ill during the 1918 flu pandemic at the same time as humans. The first influenza virus was found to be the cause of illness in pigs around 10°years later, in 1930. The World Health Organization (WHO) categorised the 2009 swine flu pandemic, which was brought on by the H1N1 influenza virus and lasted from June 2009 to August 2010, as the third recent pandemic caused by the H1N1 virus (the first being the 1918–1920 Spanish flu pandemic and the second being the 1977 Russian flu). According to two separate US investigations, the first two occurrences were discovered in April 2009. A prior triple reassortment of human, swine, and avian flu viruses combined with an additional Eurasian pig flu virus to produce what initially looked to be a novel strain of the H1N1 virus, giving rise to the term "swine flu" [29–32].

3. Structure

3.1 Corona virus composition

The lengthy RNA polymers that are tightly packed into the centre of coronavirus particles are encased in a protective capsid, which is a lattice of repeating protein molecules called the coat or capsid proteins. In coronaviruses, these proteins are referred to as nucleocapsids (N) [33, 34].

3.2 The smallpox virus's structure

The variola virus, a large double-stranded DNA pathogen with a shape akin to a brick, is serologically reactive with other members of the poxvirus family, including camel pox, vaccinia, cowpox, and ectromelia. Unlike other DNA viruses, the variola virus replicates in the cytoplasm of parasitized host cells [35, 36].

3.3 Ebola virus's structure

The Ebola virus (EBOV), a member of the family Filoviridae and genus Ebolavirus, has seven genes in its non-segmented, single-stranded RNA: (a) nucleoprotein (NP), (b) viral protein 35 (VP35), (c) VP40, (d) glycoprotein (GP), (e) VP30, (f) VP24, and (g) RNA polymerase (L) [37, 38].

3.4 The swine flu virus's structure (H1N1)

The RNA genome of the H1N1 influenza virus is around 13.5 kb in size, and its virions range in size from 80 to 120 nm. Hemagglutinin (HA) and neuraminidase, two envelope proteins (NA), are the 11 different proteins that are encoded by each of the eight segments that make up the swine influenza genome [39–41].

4. Spreading

4.1 How is the Corona virus transmitted?

When an infected person coughs, sneezes, or speaks, droplets or microscopic particles known as aerosols are emitted from their mouth or nose, dispersing the virus into the atmosphere. Anyone within 6°feet of that individual can breathe it into their lungs. Communication by air. The virus can hang about in the air for up to 3°hours, according to study [42–44].

4.2 The smallpox virus: How does it spread?

Smallpox spreads via contact with infected individuals. Smallpox is frequently spread from person to person by prolonged, direct face-to-face contact. Smallpox can also spread by contact with contaminated objects, such as contaminated bedding, clothing, or human fluids [20, 45, 46].

4.3 How does the Ebola virus circulate?

The only method to get Ebola is by direct contact with blood or other bodily fluids (such vomit, diarrhoea, urine, breast milk, sweat, or semen) from an infected person who is displaying Ebola symptoms or has recently passed away from Ebola [47, 48].

4.4 H1N1 spreads in what way?

The H1N1 virus spreads similarly to seasonal flu, according to the CDC. Droplets from an infected person's cough or sneeze, as well as touching something they recently touched and then contacting your eyes, mouth, or nose can all spread the flu [49, 50].

5. Testing

5.1 The COVID-19 test

If you are currently infected with SARS-CoV-2, the virus that causes COVID-19, a viral test will look at samples taken from your mouth or nose. The two main types of viral tests are nucleic acid amplification tests (NAATs) and antigen testing. Depending on the circumstance, one test type may be recommended over another. All tests should adhere to the FDA's regulations. A laboratory setting is used for the majority of NAATs, including PCR-based testing. They are frequently the most reliable tests, regardless of whether a person has symptoms or not. These tests identify virus genetic material, which may stay in your body for up to 90 days after a positive test result. As a result, you should not utilise an NAAT if you had a positive test within the past 90 days. Antigen test results are available in 15–30 minutes. They are less reliable than NAATs, especially for people who do not show symptoms. A single, negative antigen test result cannot exclude an infection. For the best probability of identifying infection after a negative antigen test, the test should be repeated at least 48 hours later (known as serial testing). On rare occasions, a second NAAT may be suggested to confirm the outcomes of an antigen test [6, 51, 52].

5.2 How is the small pox identified?

Smallpox can be identified based on the patient's clinical signs and symptoms. The condition can be positively identified by extracting the virus from lesions or blood and by checking for viral-specific antibodies in the blood [9, 53].

5.3 Virus testing for Ebola

After symptoms manifest, blood can be tested for the Ebola virus. Up to 3 days after the initial signs and symptoms arise, the virus may not be visible. Polymerase chain reaction (PCR) is one of the most often used diagnostic procedures because it can detect extremely low amounts of the Ebola virus [54–56].

5.4 H1N1 swine flu testing

Polymerase chain reaction (PCR) testing is becoming more common in many hospitals and labs. This test could be administered to you while you are in the hospital or at the doctor's office. PCR testing, which is more sensitive than other techniques, can be used to identify the flu strain [57–59].

6. Treatment

6.1 Treatment for COVID-19

Turn off the patient in a well-ventilated space. Utilise a triple-layered medical mask, and after 8 hours, discard it (or sooner if it becomes moist or obviously dirty). If a caregiver enters the room, the patient and the caregiver could consider donning N 95 masks. The mask must first be sterilised with 1% sodium hypochlorite before being discarded. Take a rest and drink enough of drinks to maintain proper hydration.

Always use appropriate breathing strategies. Use an alcohol-based product to disinfect your hands after regularly washing them for at least 40 seconds with soap and water. Give no access to your personal goods to family members. Ensure that a 1% hypochlorite solution is used to clean the area's commonly touched surfaces, such as tabletops, doorknobs, and handles. Check the temperature every day. To check oxygen saturation, a pulse oximeter should be used every day. Contact your medical physician right away if you notice any worsening of your symptoms [60, 61].

6.2 Treatment for smallpox

To stop an outbreak of smallpox, health officials would use vaccines. There is currently no known cure for smallpox in humans, despite the fact that some antiviral drugs may help with treatment [62, 63].

6.3 Therapy for Ebola

Delivering fluids and electrolytes (body salts) intravenously or orally (intravenously). taking medication to control fever, reduce nausea and vomiting, stabilise blood pressure, and relieve pain. Treating any further infections that may develop [64, 65].

6.4 Therapy for swine flu

Some of the antiviral drugs used to treat seasonal flu can also be used to treat H1N1 swine flu. The three antivirals zanamivir (Relenza), peramivir (Rapivab), and oseltamivir (Tamiflu) tend to be the most effective ones; nevertheless, oseltamivir is ineffective against some swine flu strains. These drugs might help you recover more quickly [32, 66].

6.5 COVID-19 vaccines vaccination

To avert this pandemic, a large segment of the population must be immune to the virus. The safest method to do this is through immunisation. In the past, vaccines have been a common method employed by humans to lessen the prevalence of infectious diseases that are lethal. A number of research teams stepped up to the plate and developed SARS-CoV-2 vaccines when the pandemic began less than a year ago. The aim now is to make these vaccines available to people everywhere. It will be vital that everyone receives the appropriate protection, not only those in wealthy countries. A COVID-19 vaccination, especially a booster, effectively protects recipients from developing severe illness, necessitating hospitalisation, and even dying. The COVID-19 vaccine is safe—much safer than getting COVID-19 from a person. People who have received the COVID-19 vaccine may benefit from additional protection from the vaccine, such as protection from having to stay in the hospital for a future infection. Similar to vaccines for other diseases, people are most protected when they receive the recommended number of doses plus boosters [67–69].

The U.S. Food and Drug Administration (FDA) has approved the smallpox vaccine ACAM2000®, (Smallpox [Vaccinia] Vaccine, Live), a replication-competent vaccine, for use in those who have been identified as having a high risk of getting smallpox. India had smallpox vaccination in 1904–1907 [70, 71].

6.6 Ebola virus illness vaccine

The Ebola Zaire Vaccine, Live, also known as V920, rVSV-G-ZEBOV-GP, or rVSV-ZEBOV, has been licenced by the U.S. Food and Drug Administration (FDA) for use in preventing Zaire ebolavirus disease in adults 18 years of age and older as a single dose administration [72–75].

6.7 Swine flu vaccine

The use of one dose of the 2009 H1N1 influenza vaccine has been authorised by the U.S. Food and Drug Administration (FDA) for people 10 years of age and older. It is recommended that children between the ages of 6 months and 9 years receive two doses of the immunisation. These two dosages should be separated by 4°weeks. The swine flu vaccine is reliable and secure. Nevertheless, a large number of people who were not at risk of contracting the virus had health problems as a result of the 1976 vaccine campaign. In contrast, the effective 2009 vaccination campaign helped to stop the H1N1 influenza pandemic in 2010 [32, 76].

7. Indian context

The primary causes of morbidity and mortality in both humans and animals continue to be infectious diseases, which has a significant financial impact on India's healthcare system. The country has had a number of epidemics and outbreaks of infectious diseases. Major epidemic diseases including cholera, leprosy, malaria, and plague have all traditionally been successfully controlled. Due to the country's varied geography, extreme geoclimatic fluctuations, and unequal population distribution, viral disease dispersion patterns are uniquely displayed. The dynamic interconnections of biological, social, and ecological variables as well as unanticipated features of the interaction between people and animals present additional challenges with regard to the origins of infectious diseases. Understanding the impact of the conditions required for the emergence and developing strengthened surveillance systems that can lessen human suffering and mortality are just two of the significant problems faced in the control and prevention of emerging and re-emerging infectious diseases. The important emerging and re-emerging viral infections of public health significance that have previously been incorporated into the Integrated Disease Surveillance Programme have been reviewed in this article.

The cholera epidemic had a significant impact on British colonial India on numerous occasions in the nineteenth century, including in the years 1817, 1829, 1852, 1863, 1881, and 1899, according to studies. Slum dwellers and the poor in rural areas, primarily in Northern Indian provinces like Punjab, Delhi, and United Provinces, made up the majority of the pandemic's casualties (current Uttar Pradesh and Uttarakhand). It gradually spread to nearby provinces, with the Madras presidency in 1877 suffering the most. Instances were noted in 1899 in Calcutta, Madras, and Bombay, three important provinces. The virus expanded to a number of countries following each epidemic, including the US, China, Arabia, Persia, and Russia. In 1992, there was a major cholera outbreak on India's southern peninsula. A cholera outbreak that followed the Orissa floods of 2001 claimed the lives of 33 individuals while infecting 34,111 others [77–79].

7.1 Smallpox (1974)

A smallpox outbreak struck West Bengal, Bihar, and Orissa in 1974. About 85% of all incidents that were reported globally were in India. In the worst smallpox pandemic of the twentieth century, around 15,000 individuals perished. Thousands of survivors suffered from blindness and deformities. The WHO launched the fight to eradicate smallpox. In 1980, the WHO deemed it extinct [80–82].

7.2 Influenza (1918–1920)

The H1N1 influenza virus caused the deadly pandemic known as the Spanish Flu or Spanish "Influenza," which claimed the lives of 20–50 million people worldwide. The flu first came in 1918, and the following year, in the fall, a second, more severe wave of the illness reappeared and swept the globe. The second wave originated in Bombay, India, and afterwards spread to Sri Lanka and the rest of the world. With an estimated death toll of 10–20 million, India served as the pandemic's mortality epicentre. One of the reasons the outbreak subsided later was the weather in India. In humid settings, the influenza virus cannot survive and cannot spread [83–85].

7.3 Polio (1970–1990)

India was affected by the polio epidemic between 1970 and 1990. India was the developing country that was most badly damaged till the late 1990s. Post-polio paralysis was widespread in children. Both urban and rural regions were severely impacted. India was the source of 40% of all polio cases that have been reported worldwide. Despite the fact that oral vaccinations were initially given there in the 1960s, India was declared polio-free in January 2011 [86].

7.4 Plague outbreaks (1994, 2002, 2004)

1994 saw a plague outbreak in Surat, Gujarat, however it was over in less than 2°weeks. The amazing panic it caused and the repercussions it had on the entire planet, nevertheless, made it noteworthy. There were only 1000 reported incidents, involving 53 fatalities. Panic and quarantine concern caused a population evacuation and internal migration [87, 88].

7.5 Encephalitis in Japan (2005)

Japanese encephalitis is a flavivirus illness that injures the brain and causes swelling that is transmitted by mosquitoes. The virus that is causing the sickness has genes in common with viruses that cause dengue and yellow fever. 2005 saw 90 occurrences in Bihar and 1145 cases from 14 districts in Uttar Pradesh. About 296 persons, or one-fourth of all those impacted, passed away. Annual reports of encephalitis cases are still common, mostly in the north (Uttar Pradesh) [89–91].

7.6 Chikungunya (2006)

In 2006, Chikungunya broke epidemic in India. Nationwide, there were almost 15 lakh recorded cases. The southern states of Gujarat, Madhya Pradesh, Maharashtra, and the Andaman and Nicobar Islands reported the majority of the cases. It was found that Aedes mosquitoes carried the illness. Chikungunya-related deaths were under-reported for a number of reasons. The outbreak was contained in part by eradicating mosquito breeding grounds, implementing additional vector control measures, promoting awareness, etc. A dengue outbreak occurred that same year, resulting in 10,344 cases and 162 fatalities [92, 93].

7.7 H1N1 flu (2010 and 2015) (2010 and 2015)

About 18,500 people died from H1N1 flu, also referred to as swine flu, in 2010. Over 27,000 confirmed cases, including 981 fatalities, were reported in India. With 30,000 cases nationally and 1731 fatalities, the flu made a comeback in 2015. The worst affected states were Gujarat, Maharashtra, and Rajasthan [94, 95].

7.8 COVID-19

India has tallied more than 18,000 confirmed cases, 600 of which have been linked to COVID-19-related fatalities. As of April 18, 2020, the COVID-19 death rate in India was 3.3%, according to the Ministry of Health. More vulnerable individuals include those who are older and/or have co-morbid disorders [96, 97].

8. Conclusions

Global social and economic conditions have been considerably disrupted by the pandemic, leading to the worst recession since the Great Depression. Supply chain instability led to widespread shortages of items, particularly food supplies. The resulting practically universal lockdowns resulted in a record-breaking decrease in emissions. The primary causes of morbidity and mortality in both humans and animals continue to be infectious diseases, which has a significant financial impact on India's healthcare system. The country has had a number of epidemics and outbreaks of infectious diseases. Major epidemic diseases including cholera, leprosy, malaria, and plague have all traditionally been successfully controlled. Due to the country's varied geography, extreme geoclimatic fluctuations, and unequal population distribution, viral disease dispersion patterns are uniquely displayed. The dynamic interconnections of biological, social, and ecological variables as well as unanticipated features of the interaction between people and animals present additional challenges with regard to the origins of infectious diseases. Two of the major challenges in the control and prevention of emerging and re-emerging infectious diseases are understanding the effects of the conditions necessary for their emergence and creating strengthened surveillance systems that can reduce human misery and mortality. This article reviews the significant emerging and re-emerging viral illnesses of public health importance that have previously been included in the Integrated Disease Surveillance Programme. India is always at danger from newly emerging and re-emerging viral infections that are important for public health because of its great geoclimatic variety. With an emphasis on epidemiology and disease burden, illness surveillance needs to be strengthened across the country. In-depth knowledge of disease biology, particularly that of disease vectors and the effects of the environment on disease, is also urgently needed. It is also necessary to increase emergency preparedness for these diseases and response by focusing on the "one health" idea. India had a gradual rise in the number of cases after the first case was identified on January 30, 2020. However, given that testing approach and skills have progressively improved, India's meagre testing efforts may reflect an underestimate of COVID-19 circumstances. Additionally, the clear selective policy of only screening symptomatic individuals contributed to the under-representation of the genuine case counts. This brought to light the fact that there are incidences in India that go unreported. It is essential to develop a universal testing method for all symptomatic, asymptomatic, pre-symptomatic, and post-symptomatic cases in order to successfully stop the spread of COVID-19, which is on the rise. Given its vast population and high danger of community transmission, this is particularly true in India. India uses the corona virus spike proteins to represent different COVID-19 defence systems (**Figure 1**). To combat COVID-19, the Indian government has undertaken a number of activities, including testing, vaccination, mask and sanitizer use, genome sequencing, government and public awareness campaigns, research, and the improvement of health infrastructure. With the aid of a large number of tests, including RT-PCR and rapid antigen testing kits, India's indigenous COVID-19 vaccine COVAXIN, developed by Bharat Biotech in collaboration with the Indian Council of Medical Research (ICMR) - National Institute of Virology (NIV), and the vaccine Covishield manufactured and large-scale production by the Serum Institute of India, played a significant role in inhibiting the rapid spread of the pandemic (UK). There was a severe shortage of masks and sanitizers during the COVID-19's initial phase, but internal production, large-scale production, and distribution severely damaged the chain. Genome sequencing in India occasionally helped to detect the different altered Corona virus strains. In India, public awareness campaigns and government regulations were key in preventing the COVID-19 virus from spreading. For the COVID-19, which included research labs, institutes, and universities all over India, researchers

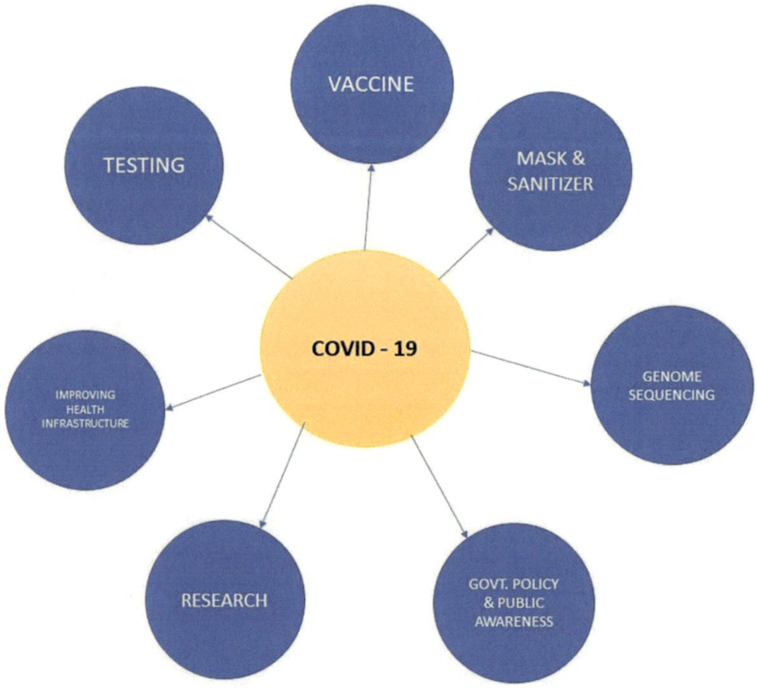

Figure 1.
Different strategies for COVID-19 in India represented as spike proteins of Corona virus.

worked tirelessly to oversee the Research and Development units. Instead of India's underdeveloped healthcare infrastructure, ongoing work is being done to create appropriate facilities with proper management of healthcare infrastructure, such as converting regular hospitals into COVID-19 hospitals that are specially outfitted and redesigned to meet the needs of patients infected with the virus.

Author details

Aishwarya Khamari[1*], Monika Khamari[2], Akshya Kumar Mishra[3], Jijnasa Panda[1], Debashish Gardia[4] and Ratikanta Rath[5]

1 School of Life Sciences, Sambalpur University, Sambalpur, India

2 Department of Biotechnology and Bioinformatics, Sambalpur University, Sambalpur, India

3 Department of Microbiology, Batakrushna College of Pharmacy, Nuapada, India

4 Department of Pharmacology, Batakrushna College of Pharmacy, Nuapada, India

5 Department of Zoology, Government Women's College Sambalpur, Sambalpur, India

*Address all correspondence to: khamariaishwarya@gmail.com

References

[1] Khan M, Adil SF, Alkhathlan HZ, Tahir MN, Saif S, Khan M, et al. COVID-19: A global challenge with old history, epidemiology and progress so far. Molecules. 2020;**26**(1):39

[2] Evans L, Rhodes A, Alhazzani W, Antonelli M, Coopersmith CM, French C, et al. Surviving sepsis campaign: International guidelines for management of sepsis and septic shock 2021. Intensive Care Medicine. 2021;**47**(11):1181-1247

[3] Azoulay E, De Waele J, Ferrer R, Staudinger T, Borkowska M, Povoa P, et al. Symptoms of burnout in intensive care unit specialists facing the COVID-19 outbreak. Annals of Intensive Care. 2020;**10**(1):1-8

[4] Mertens G, Duijndam S, Smeets T, Lodder P. The latent and item structure of COVID-19 fear: A comparison of four COVID-19 fear questionnaires using SEM and network analyses. Journal of Anxiety Disorders. 2021;**81**:102415

[5] Vos LM, Habibović M, Nyklíček I, Smeets T, Mertens G. Optimism, mindfulness, and resilience as potential protective factors for the mental health consequences of fear of the coronavirus. Psychiatry Research. 2021;**300**:113927

[6] Mercer TR, Salit M. Testing at scale during the COVID-19 pandemic. Nature Reviews Genetics. 2021;**22**(7):415-426

[7] Wong DW, Li Y. Spreading of COVID-19: Density matters. PLoS One. 2020;**15**(12):e0242398

[8] Kalantar-Zadeh K, Ward SA, Kalantar-Zadeh K, El-Omar EM. Considering the effects of microbiome and diet on SARS-CoV-2 infection: Nanotechnology roles. ACS Nano. 2020;**14**(5):5179-5182

[9] Peeling RW, Wedderburn CJ, Garcia PJ, Boeras D, Fongwen N, Nkengasong J, et al. Serology testing in the COVID-19 pandemic response. The Lancet Infectious Diseases. 2020;**20**(9):e245-e249

[10] Hrusak O, Kalina T, Wolf J, Balduzzi A, Provenzi M, Rizzari C, et al. Flash survey on severe acute respiratory syndrome coronavirus-2 infections in paediatric patients on anticancer treatment. European Journal of Cancer. 2020;**132**:11-16

[11] Manabe YC, Sharfstein JS, Armstrong K. The need for more and better testing for COVID-19. Jama. 2020;**324**(21):2153-2154

[12] Binnicker MJ. Challenges and controversies to testing for COVID-19. Journal of Clinical Microbiology. 2020;**58**(11):e01695-e01620

[13] Gautret P, Million M, Jarrot PA, Camoin-Jau L, Colson P, Fenollar F, et al. Natural history of COVID-19 and therapeutic options. Expert Review of Clinical Immunology. 2020;**16**(12):1159-1184

[14] Dos Santos WG. Natural history of COVID-19 and current knowledge on treatment therapeutic options. Biomedicine and Pharmacotherapy. 2020;**129**:110493

[15] Balkhair AA. COVID-19 pandemic: A new chapter in the history of infectious diseases. Oman Medical Journal. 2020;**35**(2):e123

[16] Jones DS. History in a crisis—Lessons for Covid-19. New England Journal of Medicine. 2020;**382**(18):1681-1683

[17] Ferrer R. COVID-19 pandemic: The greatest challenge in the history of critical care. Medicina Intensiva. 2020;**44**(6):323

[18] Geddes AM. The history of smallpox. Clinics in Dermatology. 2006;**24**(3):152-157

[19] Riedel S. Edward Jenner and the history of smallpox and vaccination. In: Baylor University Medical Center Proceedings. Vol. 18, 1. Taylor & Francis; January 2005. pp. 21-25

[20] Thèves C, Crubézy E, Biagini P. History of smallpox and its spread in human populations. Microbiology Spectrum. 2016;**4**(4):4-4

[21] Duggan AT, Perdomo MF, Piombino-Mascali D, Marciniak S, Poinar D, Emery MV, et al. 17th century variola virus reveals the recent history of smallpox. Current Biology. 2016;**26**(24):3407-3412

[22] Fenner F, Henderson DA, Arita I, Jezek Z, Ladnyi ID. The history of smallpox and its spread around the world. Smallpox and its Eradication. 1988:209-244

[23] Huerkamp C. The history of smallpox vaccination in Germany: A first step in the medicalization of the general public. Journal of Contemporary History. 1985;**20**(4):617-635

[24] Pourrut X, Kumulungui B, Wittmann T, Moussavou G, Délicat A, Yaba P, et al. The natural history of Ebola virus in Africa. Microbes and Infection. 2005;7(7-8):1005-1014

[25] Li YH, Chen SP. Evolutionary history of Ebola virus. Epidemiology and Infection. 2014;**142**(6):1138-1145

[26] Majid MU, Tahir MS, Ali Q, Rao AQ, Rashid B, Ali A, et al. Nature and history of Ebola virus: An overview. Archives of Neuroscience. 2016;**3**(3)

[27] Weyer J, Grobbelaar A, Blumberg L. Ebola virus disease: History, epidemiology and outbreaks. Current Infectious Disease Reports. 2015;**17**(5):1-8

[28] Murray MJ. Ebola virus disease: A review of its past and present. Anesthesia and Analgesia. 2015;**121**(3):798-809

[29] Mir SA, Tandon VR, Abbas Z, Singh Z, Farhat S, Pukhta MA, et al. History of swine flu. JK Science. 2009;**11**(4):163

[30] Berridge V, Taylor S. The problems of commissioned oral history: The swine flu 'crisis' of 2009. Oral History. 2019:86-94

[31] Schultz-Cherry S, Olsen CW, Easterday BC. History of swine influenza. Swine Influenza. 2011:21-27

[32] Parmar S, Shah N, Kasarwala M, Virpura M, Prajapati DD. A review on swine flu. Journal of Pharmaceutical Science and Bioscientific Research. 2011;**1**(1):11-17

[33] Dumar AM. Swine Flu: What you Need to Know. Wildside Press LLC; 2009

[34] Zeng Q, Langereis MA, Van Vliet AL, Huizinga EG, De Groot RJ. Structure of coronavirus hemagglutinin-esterase offers insight into corona and influenza virus evolution. Proceedings of the National Academy of Sciences. 2008;**105**(26):9065-9069

[35] Brian DA, Baric RS. Coronavirus genome structure and replication. Coronavirus Replication and Reverse Genetics. 2005:1-30

[36] Perry K, Hwang Y, Bushman FD, Van Duyne GD. Insights from the structure of a smallpox virus topoisomerase-DNA

transition state mimic. Structure. 2010;**18**(1):127-137

[37] Lee JE, Fusco ML, Hessell AJ, Oswald WB, Burton DR, Saphire EO. Structure of the Ebola virus glycoprotein bound to an antibody from a human survivor. Nature. 2008;**454**(7201):177-182

[38] Wan W, Kolesnikova L, Clarke M, Koehler A, Noda T, Becker S, et al. Structure and assembly of the Ebola virus nucleocapsid. Nature. 2017;**551**(7680):394-397

[39] Pallesen J, Murin CD, De Val N, Cottrell CA, Hastie KM, Turner HL, et al. Structures of Ebola virus GP and sGP in complex with therapeutic antibodies. Nature Microbiology. 2016;**1**(9):1-9

[40] Soundararajan V, Tharakaraman K, Raman R, Raguram S, Shriver Z, Sasisekharan V, et al. Extrapolating from sequence—The 2009 H1N1'swine'influenza virus. Nature Biotechnology. 2009;**27**(6):510-513

[41] Wentworth DE, Thompson BL, Xu XIYAN, Regnery HL, Cooley AJ, McGregor MW, et al. An influenza A (H1N1) virus, closely related to swine influenza virus, responsible for a fatal case of human influenza. Journal of Virology. 1994;**68**(4):2051-2058

[42] Xu R, Ekiert DC, Krause JC, Hai R, Crowe JE Jr, Wilson IA. Structural basis of preexisting immunity to the 2009 H1N1 pandemic influenza virus. Science. 2010;**328**(5976):357-360

[43] Khan N, Fahad S. Critical review of the present situation of corona virus in China. 2020. Available at SSRN 3543177

[44] Din A, Li Y, Khan T, Zaman G. Mathematical analysis of spread and control of the novel corona virus (COVID-19) in China. Chaos, Solitons & Fractals. 2020;**141**:110286

[45] Mesgarpour M, Abad JMN, Alizadeh R, Wongwises S, Doranehgard MH, Ghaderi S, et al. Prediction of the spread of Corona-virus carrying droplets in a bus-a computational based artificial intelligence approach. Journal of Hazardous Materials. 2021;**413**:125358

[46] Reynolds MG, Carroll DS, Karem KL. Factors affecting the likelihood of monkeypox's emergence and spread in the post-smallpox era. Current Opinion in Virology. 2012;**2**(3):335-343

[47] Ferguson NM, Keeling MJ, John Edmunds W, Gani R, Grenfell BT, Anderson RM, et al. Planning for smallpox outbreaks. Nature. 2003;**425**(6959):681-685

[48] Dixon MG, Schafer IJ. Ebola viral disease outbreak—West Africa, 2014. Morbidity and Mortality Weekly Report. 2014;**63**(25):548

[49] Holmes EC, Dudas G, Rambaut A, Andersen KG. The evolution of Ebola virus: Insights from the 2013-2016 epidemic. Nature. 2016;**538**(7624):193-200

[50] Khan K, Arino J, Hu W, Raposo P, Sears J, Calderon F, et al. Spread of a novel influenza A (H1N1) virus via global airline transportation. New England Journal of Medicine. 2009;**361**(2):212-214

[51] López-Cervantes M, Venado A, Moreno A, Pacheco-Domínguez RL, Ortega-Pierres G. On the spread of the novel influenza a (H1N1) virus in Mexico. The Journal of Infection in Developing Countries. 2009;**3**(05):327-330

[52] Beeching NJ, Fletcher TE, Beadsworth MB. Covid-19: Testing times. BMJ. 2020;**369**

[53] Breman JG, Henderson DA. Diagnosis and management of smallpox.

New England Journal of Medicine. 2002;**346**(17):1300-1308

[54] O'Toole T. Smallpox: An attack scenario. Emerging Infectious Diseases. 1999;**5**(4):540

[55] Broadhurst MJ, Brooks TJ, Pollock NR. Diagnosis of Ebola virus disease: Past, present, and future. Clinical Microbiology Reviews. 2016;**29**(4):773-793

[56] Katz LM, Tobian AA. Ebola virus disease, transmission risk to laboratory personnel, and pretransfusion testing. Transfusion. 2014;**54**(12):3247-3251

[57] World Health Organization. Clinical Care for Survivors of Ebola Virus Disease: Interim Guidance (No. WHO/EVD/OHE/PED/16.1 Rev. 2). World Health Organization; 2016

[58] Burkardt HJ. Pandemic H1N1 2009 ('swine flu'): Diagnostic and other challenges. Expert Review of Molecular Diagnostics. 2011;**11**(1):35-40

[59] Faix DJ, Sherman SS, Waterman SH. Rapid-test sensitivity for novel swine-origin influenza a (H1N1) virus in humans. New England Journal of Medicine. 2009;**361**(7):728-729

[60] Chauhan N, Narang J, Pundir S, Singh S, Pundir CS. Laboratory diagnosis of swine flu: A review. Artificial cells, Nanomedicine, and Biotechnology. 2013;**41**(3):189-195

[61] Stasi C, Fallani S, Voller F, Silvestri C. Treatment for COVID-19: An overview. European Journal of Pharmacology. 2020;**889**:173644

[62] Joshi S, Parkar J, Ansari A, Vora A, Talwar D, Tiwaskar M, et al. Role of favipiravir in the treatment of COVID-19. International Journal of Infectious Diseases. 2021;**102**:501-508

[63] Melamed S, Israely T, Paran N. Challenges and achievements in prevention and treatment of smallpox. Vaccine. 2018;**6**(1):8

[64] Grosenbach DW, Honeychurch K, Rose EA, Chinsangaram J, Frimm A, Maiti B, et al. Oral tecovirimat for the treatment of smallpox. New England Journal of Medicine. 2018;**379**(1):44-53

[65] Bixler SL, Duplantier AJ, Bavari S. Discovering drugs for the treatment of Ebola virus. Current Treatment Options in Infectious Diseases. 2017;**9**(3):299-317

[66] Zarocostas J. WHO recommends early antiviral treatment for at risk groups with suspected swine flu. BMJ: British Medical Journal (Online). 2009;**339**

[67] Biswas N, Mustapha T, Khubchandani J, Price JH. The nature and extent of COVID-19 vaccination hesitancy in healthcare workers. Journal of Community Health. 2021;**46**(6):1244-1251

[68] DeRoo SS, Pudalov NJ, Fu LY. Planning for a COVID-19 vaccination program. JAMA. 2020;**323**(24):2458-2459

[69] Sherman SM, Smith LE, Sim J, Amlôt R, Cutts M, Dasch H, et al. COVID-19 vaccination intention in the UK: Results from the COVID-19 vaccination acceptability study (CoVAccS), a nationally representative cross-sectional survey. Human Vaccines & Immunotherapeutics. 2021;**17**(6):1612-1621

[70] Belongia EA, Naleway AL. Smallpox vaccine: The good, the bad, and the ugly. Clinical Medicine & Research. 2003;**1**(2):87-92

[71] Parrino J, Graham BS. Smallpox vaccines: Past, present, and future. Journal of Allergy and Clinical Immunology. 2006;**118**(6):1320-1326

[72] Tomori O, Kolawole MO. Ebola virus disease: Current vaccine solutions. Current Opinion in Immunology. 2021;**71**:27-33

[73] Ohimain EI. Recent advances in the development of vaccines for Ebola virus disease. Virus Research. 2016;**211**:174-185

[74] Lévy Y, Lane C, Piot P, Beavogui AH, Kieh M, Leigh B, et al. Prevention of Ebola virus disease through vaccination: Where we are in 2018. The Lancet. 2018;**392**(10149):787-790

[75] Kennedy SB, Neaton JD, Lane HC, Kieh MW, Massaquoi MB, Touchette NA, et al. Implementation of an Ebola virus disease vaccine clinical trial during the Ebola epidemic in Liberia: Design, procedures, and challenges. Clinical Trials. 2016;**13**(1):49-56

[76] Carlsen B, Glenton C. The swine flu vaccine, public attitudes, and researcher interpretations: A systematic review of qualitative research. BMC Health Services Research. 2016;**16**(1):1-15

[77] Briggs A. Cholera and society in the nineteenth century. Past and Present. 1961;**19**:76-96

[78] Klein I. Imperialism, ecology and disease: Cholera in India, 1850-1950. The Indian Economic and Social History Review. 1994;**31**(4):491-518

[79] Huber V. Pandemics and the politics of difference: Rewriting the history of internationalism through nineteenth-century cholera. Journal of Global History. 2020;**15**(3):394-407

[80] Mukherjee MK, Sarkar JK, Mitra AC. Pattern of intrafamilial transmission of smallpox in Calcutta, India. Bulletin of the World Health Organization. 1974;**51**(3):219

[81] Morinis EA. Tapping the flow of information in a rural region: The example of the smallpox eradication program in Bihar, India. Human Organization. 1980;**39**(2):180-184

[82] Jezek Z, Das MN, Das A, Arya ZS, World Health Organization. The Last Known Outbreak of Smallpox in India (No. WHO/SE/76.84). World Health Organization; 1976

[83] Chandra S, Kassens-Noor E. The evolution of pandemic influenza: Evidence from India, 1918-19. BMC Infectious Diseases. 2014;**14**(1):1-10

[84] Hill K. Influenza in India 1918: Excess mortality reassessed. Genus. 2011;**67**(2):9-29

[85] Athukorala P, Athukorala C. The Great Influenza Pandemic of 1918-20: An Interpretative Survey in the Time of COVID-19 (No. 2020/124). WIDER Working Paper. 2020

[86] John TJ, Vashishtha VM. Eradicating poliomyelitis: India's journey from hyperendemic to polio-free status. The Indian Journal of Medical Research. 2013;**137**(5):881

[87] Deodhar NS, Yemul VL, Banerjee K. Plague that never was: A review of the alleged plague outbreaks in India in 1994. Journal of Public Health Policy. 1998;**19**(2):184-199

[88] Clem A, Galwankar S. Plague: A decade since the 1994 outbreaks in India. The Journal of the Association of Physicians of India. 2005;**53**:457-464

[89] Parida M, Dash PK, Tripathi NK, Sannarangaiah S, Saxena P, Agarwal S, et al. Japanese encephalitis outbreak, India, 2005. Emerging Infectious Diseases. 2006;**12**(9):1427

[90] Kabilan L, Rajendran R, Arunachalam N, Ramesh S, Srinivasan S, Samuel PP, et al. Japanese encephalitis in India: An overview. The Indian Journal of Pediatrics. 2004;**71**(7):609-615

[91] Kumari R, Joshi PL. A review of Japanese encephalitis in Uttar Pradesh, India. WHO South-East Asia Journal of Public Health. 2012;**1**(4):374-395

[92] Tandale BV, Sathe PS, Arankalle VA, Wadia RS, Kulkarni R, Shah SV, et al. Systemic involvements and fatalities during chikungunya epidemic in India, 2006. Journal of Clinical Virology. 2009;**46**(2):145-149

[93] Cecilia D. Current status of dengue and chikungunya in India. WHO South-East Asia Journal of Public Health. 2014;**3**(1):22

[94] Rathi SK. Knowledge and awareness about H1N1 flu in urban adult population of Vadodara, India: Array. Electronic Physician. 2011;**3**(1):392-395

[95] Chawla R, Sharma RK, Bhardwaj JR. Influenza a (H1N1) outbreak and challenges for pharmacotherapy. Indian Journal of Physiology and Pharmacology. 2009;**53**(2):113-126

[96] Das M, Das A, Mandal A. Examining the impact of lockdown (due to COVID-19) on domestic violence (DV): An evidences from India. Asian Journal of Psychiatry. 2020;**54**:102335

[97] Mishra P, Fatih C, Rawat D, Sahu S, Pandey SA, Ray M, et al. Trajectory of COVID-19 data in India: Investigation and project using artificial neural network, fuzzy time series and ARIMA models. Annual Research and Review in Biology. 2020:46-54

Section 3

Viral Outbreaks Linked to Animals

Chapter 6

Leporids' Emerging Diseases as a Threat to Biodiversity

Fábio A. Abade dos Santos, Teresa Fagulha, Sílvia S. Barros, Margarida Henriques, Ana Duarte, Fernanda Ramos, Tiago Luís and Margarida D. Duarte

Abstract

Wild leporids have been gaining interest and prominence in the scientific and social community worldwide. While endangered of extinction in its native territory, the Iberian Peninsula, where it has a key role in the Mediterranean ecosystems, the European rabbit (*Oryctolagus cuniculus*) is considered a plague in Australia, due to the great economic and ecological consequences of its presence in the territories. The impact of viral diseases on the Leporidae family' members, namely on the European rabbit, has been largely recognized worldwide since the early 50s, due to the emergence of myxomatosis and, from the mid-80s onwards, due to the emergence of rabbit haemorrhagic disease virus 1 and 2. More recently, in 2018, a recombinant myxoma virus emerged with the ability to infect and cause severe disease in the Iberian hare (*Lepus ganatensis*). Also, a new gammaherpesvirus was described in Iberian hares, associated with myxoma virus infections. In this chapter, we revise the main viral infectious treats to the native leporids of the Iberian Peninsula. The recovery of the European rabbit populations, as well as of other leporid species around the world, is currently a major challenge for the scientific and social communities and policy-makers. If we fail, the ripple effects on the trophic web will be so dramatic that are likely to be unrecoverable.

Keywords: wild leporids, viral treats, European rabbit, Iberian hare, myxomatosis, rabbit haemorrhagic disease, endangered species

1. Introduction

With the earliest known fossil ancestor identified in Mongolia 55 million years ago [1], Leporidae is the biggest family of order Lagomorpha and includes rabbits and hares (and also the jackrabbits), divided into 11 genera comprising 62 species, characterized, among other features, for the 28 teeth (incisor 2/1, canine 0/0, premolar 3/2, molar 3/3) (**Figure 1**) [2].

Together with family Ochotonidae that includes the pikas, Leporidae family constitute the mammalian Lagomorpha order. The 11 genera within the Leporidae family comprise genus *Caprolagus* (1 species), genus *Lepus* (32 species), genus *Pronolagus*

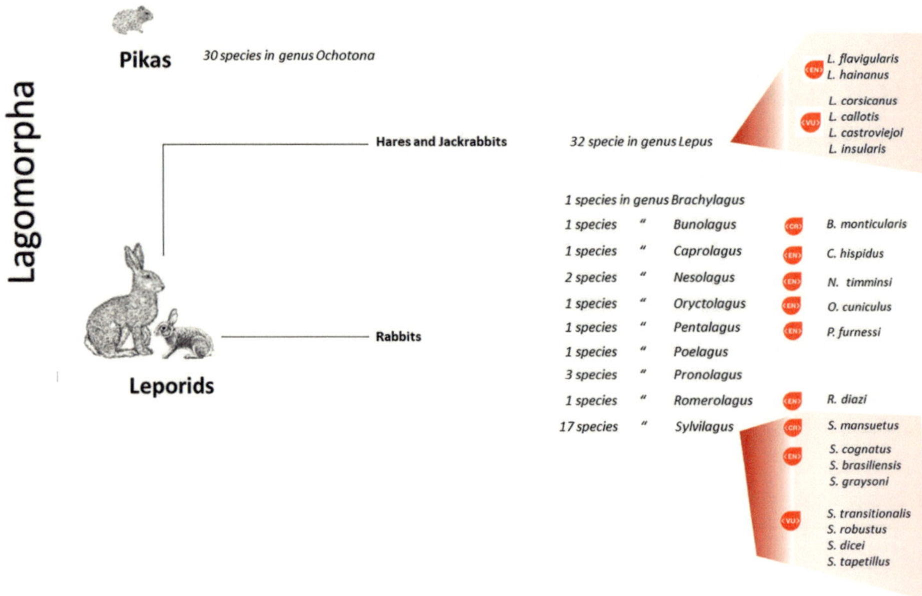

Figure 1.
Genera in families Ochotonidae (pikas) and Leporidae (leporids). The scientific names of species with conservation status of vulnerable, threatened or critically endangered by the IUCN are presented.

(3 species), genus *Sylvilagus* (17 species), genus *Brachylagus* (1 species), genus *Bunolagus* (1 species), genus *Nesolagus* (1 species), genus *Oryctolagus* (1 species), genus *Pentalagus* (1 species), genus *Poelagus* (1 species) and genus *Romerolagus* (1 species).

Except for Antarctica and Australia, all continents have indigenous species of Leporidae. Genus *Lepus* is the most speciose genus and has a worldwide distribution [3], despite only six of these species inhabit Europe.

The European rabbit was introduced to most of Oceania as to other islands. The European rabbit, *Oryctolagus cuniculus* (Linnaeus, 1958), is native to the Iberian Peninsula and the south of France, while genus *Sylvilagus* is widely distributed across North, Central and South America, although most species are confined to specific regions.

Twelve species, namely 11 from *Lepus* genus and the European rabbit, have seen their geographic distribution expanded by human translocations since the year 1400 BC [4].

Leporids are key species in many ecosystems [5, 6] due to their role as primary consumers transforming the vegetal protein in high-quality animal protein [7–9], impacting directly and indirectly in the ecosystems. Its variable weight range, from *Oryctolagus cuniculus algirus* with less than 1 kg to *Lepus europaeus* with ~5 kg of weight, offers the ideal biomass intake for many predators from small, such as the genet, to big sizes, such as the lynx and eagles.

The reduction of native species can cause important changes in the structure and function of natural ecosystems affecting directly its intermediate and top predators, and indirectly other species belonging to the same and other linked web chains.

Regarding their behaviour, rabbits and hares are crepuscular, being most active at sunrise and sunset, during the twilight hours, being ideal prey species for predators with the same habits.

In native countries, these species have a huge impact on plant community composition and dissemination, slowing down some invasive grass species. However, in some cases, wild leporids have a great impact in the recruitment of young trees, forest restoration and maintenance of important native vegetation, while still having a positive impact on the survival of plants in hostile environments, being important in both mechanisms of endozoochory or epizoochory [10–13].

European rabbit (*O. cuniculus*) is the most paradigmatic and well-studied leporid being a endemic species of Iberian Peninsula, consumed by more than 40 terrestrial and aerial carnivore species providing the primary biomass source for many of them [14–16], namely the paradigmatic Iberian lynx and Spanish Imperial eagle that include wild rabbits in about 90% of the diet [17]. Leporids are even preyed upon by very unusual predators, from light-weight terrestrial birds, such as the Greater Roadrunner (*Geococcyx californianus*) or the American red squirrel (*Tamiasciurus hudsonicus*) [18, 19].

High abundances of *O. cuniculus* may also have cascading effects by promoting the presence of top predators, such as the Iberian lynx, which regulate mesopredators, such as the Egyptian mongoose, *Herpestes ichneumon*, either *via* intraguild predation or by consuming their main prey [20].

The impacts of European rabbit in the Iberian Peninsula (Portugal and Spain) are the most notorious and well-studied, taking into account the essential effects of wild rabbit on these territories. Belonging to one of the 34 global ecological hotspots—the western corner of the Mediterranean Basin hotspot—second only to the tropics in importance [21], Iberia contains the same plant richness (30,000 taxa) of all tropical Africa (four times larger) and 10.8 species/1000 km^2, higher than China, Zaira, India and Brazil [22]. The reduction of leporids in this type of rich territories has brutal knock-on effects with tropic cascades, leading to threatens to all the trophic chains [16, 23]. The deregulation of the trophic chain also leads to the deregulation of the biomass sources of predators with effects on the proximity of predators to humans and with an increase in conflicting events between fauna and man. The principal events of viral threats are shown in the **Figure 2**.

Many factors account for the abrupt reduction of wild leporids in the last decades including habitat loss to agriculture or intensive forest regimes, habitat disturbance and fragmentation, intensification of agriculture with monoculture farming, excessive hunting pressure, excessive predation, climate exchanges (thermal limits, vegetation, rainfall) and soil type (impacting on burrowing and growing of major food species) [16, 24, 25]. In fact, all these parameters insidiously and chronically influence the wild rabbit populations, which are then subject to epidemic outbreaks, more visible and better studied, of various diseases, particularly those of viral aetiology.

Paradoxically, European rabbit (*O. cuniculus*) is also included on the '100 of the world's worst invasive alien species' list, and much scientific attention has been paid to this species as it has led to significant economic and ecological losses [26, 27].

Their high reproduction rates may be their main strategy to cope with predation, which in some cases can cause juvenile mortality of up to 90% [28, 29]. Most leporids have multiple litters per year, with litter sizes varying from 1 to 11 individuals, and each female producing between 10 and 45 young per year [6, 30, 31].

The presence of leporid species can also constitute a human-wildlife health hazard, as they act as natural reservoirs of many zoonotic diseases including, among many others, tularaemia, Lyme borreliosis and Crimean-Congo haemorrhagic fever [32].

In Argentinean Patagonia, the prevalence of *Fasciola hepatica* in *L. europaeus* is sufficient to maintain a viable wild reservoir of this disease [33, 34]. *Sylvilagus floridanus* is an effective vector of the West Nile virus, a threat to several vertebrate species [35], mainly human, horses and birds, and carries dermatophyte fungi that affect humans [36]. In its exotic geographic range in Italy, *S. floridanus* hosts many transmittable parasites and is an asymptomatic carrier of myxomatosis and pseudotuberculosis, directly affecting native leporids [37].

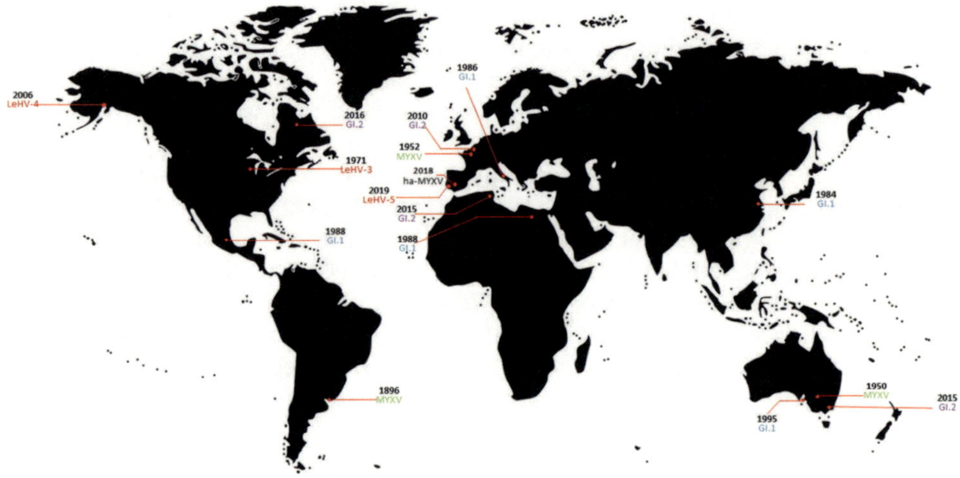

Figure 2.
Major virus emergencies impacting wild leporids. LeHV, leporid herpesvirus; MYXV, myxoma virus; ha-MYXV, natural recombinant myxoma virus; GI.1, Lagovirus europaeus genogroup I, genotype 1 (RHDV); GI.2, Lagovirus europaeus genogroup I, genotype 2 (RHDV2/RHDVb).

As obligatory intracellular parasites, viruses have evolved and adapted to their hosts in order to survive and produce a viable progeny. To do so, viruses need to take over the cellular metabolism from which they are totally dependent. Highly complex viruses, such as myxoma virus, can evade the host defence mechanisms by modulating the immune response through viral proteins.

In most occasions, viruses cause asymptomatic subclinical or mild infections in their natural hosts (reservoirs), a way to guarantee a continuous source and spread of virus for new replication cycles. Viral infections tend to be less aggressive in their natural host species, to which viruses are well adapted, than in introduced species, with no history of contact with (and adaptation to) the virus [38]. A good example of this is provided by myxoma virus, which produces a small benign fibroma in its natural host the *Sylvilagus* spp., the American rabbit (myxoma virus natural host or reservoir), but a highly pathogenic disease in the European rabbit (*Oryctolagus cuniculus*).

In some situations, viruses can infect other species, previously unknown to be susceptible to the infection, an event of cross-species transmission. This may be a rare finding, as it was the report of RHDV2 in Iberian hare in Spain [39], designated a spillover event, with no apparent consequences, or, on the contrary, may lead to severe infection in the new host. This is well exemplified by the emergence of a new recombinant myxoma virus (ha-MYXV) that acquired the capacity to infect Iberian hares, causing high mortality.

Identifying the viruses' reservoirs provides crucial information for the knowledge of the epidemiology of the infections and the potential for transmission to other hosts. While MYXV reservoir is well known, RHDV2 reservoir is still unknown, despite some wild species, such as the Eurasian badger, are possible candidates.

2. Viral threats

Although the susceptibility of pikas to some viral agents such as Influenza [40] or Coronavirus [41] is recognized, to date no disease has been described that assumes great significance in terms of morbidity and mortality in this family, so they will not be described below.

2.1 Leporipoxviruses (MYXV, ha-MYXV and RFV)

2.1.1 Taxonomic classification

Leporipoxviruses affects mainly leporids and belong to *Chordopoxvirinae* subfamily, within *Poxviridae* family.

The following leporipoxviruses [42] and respective natural hosts are presently known:

a. Myxoma virus—Tapeti (*Sylvilagus brasiliensis*)

b. Californian myxoma virus—Brush rabbit (*Sylvilagus bachmani*)

c. Rabbit (Shope) fibroma virus—Eastern cottontail (*Sylvilagus floridanus*)

d. Squirrel fibroma virus—Eastern grey squirrel (*Sciurus carolinensis*)

e. Hare fibroma virus—European brown hare (*Lepus europaeus*)

f. Western squirrel fibroma virus—Western grey squirrel (*Sciurus griseus griseus*)

2.1.2 Morphology and genome organization

The MYXV strain Lausanne (Lu), Brazil/Campinas 1949, considered *de facto* the international reference strain (ATCC code VR-115), has a double-stranded DNA (dsDNA) genome with 161,777 bp of size and closed single-strand hairpin termini. The genome encodes a total of 158 ORFs with 12 duplicates in the 577 bp terminal inverted repeats (TIRs) [43, 44]. The viral genome is encapsidated in a brick-shaped virion, and the replication cycle occurs in the cytoplasm of infected cells where a spectrum of host-interactive immunomodulatory proteins is expressed [45].

Genes-encoding proteins involved in replication and structure are relatively conserved among other poxviruses and tend to be located in the central part of the genome, while genes at the termini of the genome tend to encode host-range and virulence factors [44, 46]. The function of 42 viral genes is related to the host range or immunomodulation [47].

2.1.3 Viral replication

The most well-studied intracellular replication cycle concerns vaccinia virus (VV). Both the intracellular mature virus (IMV) and the extracellular enveloped virus (EEV), which differ in their surface glycoproteins and in the number of layer membranes, can initiate the infectious cycle, using different mechanisms [48].

Poxvirus replication cycle begins with binding of the virus to the cell surface, probably ubiquitously expressed glycosaminoglycans or components of the extracellular matrix, triggering signalling events in several host protein-kinase cascades [48]. Subsequently, fusion of the virus envelope with the mammalian cell membranes occurs, with release of the virion core structure into the cytoplasm [48].

Once the virus core has been released into the cytoplasm, the cellular RNA polymerase and the encapsidated transcription factors initiate the first round of early viral gene expression, which synthesizes viral mRNA under the control of viral early promoters [49, 50]. Then, core uncoating releases the viral DNA into the cytoplasm, where it serves as template for DNA replication and for subsequent events of intermediate and late transcription, where host-derived transcription factors participate. As late viral gene products accumulate, progressive morphogenesis and assembly of infectious virus particles take place, initially as IMV virions, which assemble and migrate *via* microtubules being wrapped with Golgi-derived membranes to form intracellular enveloped virus (IEV) [48].

2.1.4 Epidemiology (origin, transmission and distribution)

Myxoma virus (MYXV)—reference virus, Rabbit fibroma virus (RFV) and more recently the natural recombinant myxoma virus (ha-MYXV or rec-MYXV) are the three poxviruses that most impact on leporids. Brazilian cottontail is the natural host of MYXV, while Eastern cottontail rabbit (*S. floridanus*) is the natural host of RFV, with both viruses causing benign and non-fatal infections in these hosts. On the contrary, in the European rabbit (*O. cuniculus*), RFV causes skin tumours (myxomas) with benign progression and MYXV causes impacting disease (named myxomatosis), generally lethal.

Until recently, MYXV infected only rabbits and European brown hares (*L. europaeus*), the last species only occasionally with clinical signs [51–53]. Apart from lagomorphs, MYXV is non-pathogenic for any of the hosts tested so far [52].

Myxomatosis was first described in 1896 in Montevideo, Uruguay, following the acquisition of European rabbit (*O. cuniculus*) for antiserum production [54]. The origin of the virus was attributed to the Eastern cottontail rabbit. After the disease being described, myxoma virus would come to be introduced by man in Chile (Tierra del Fuego), France and Australia [51, 55, 56] to control the extremely large rabbit populations, considered a plague, with excellent results in the short term but not effective in the medium and long term. The unsuccess of biological control happened again over time, either through the selection of less pathogenic virus strains or through the genetic selection of more resistant rabbits [42, 57, 58].

2.1.5 Pathogenesis and disease characterization

The replication of MYXV inoculated intradermally in European rabbit initiates in MHC-II+ cells at the dermal/epidermal interface. Then, the virus spreads to the draining lymph node, first replicating in cells of the subcapsular sinus and later in lymphocytes of T cell zones. Lymphocytes, and possibly monocytes, disseminate the virus to distal tissues, with low viral load detectable in the bloodstream [59–61]. Simultaneously, in the original inoculation site, the virus replicates in epidermal cells inducing hyperplasia and hypertrophy, disrupting the dermis and causing oedema and infiltration of mucoid material in the sub-dermis matrix—originating the myxoid tissue that is responsible for the virus's name. The epidermal cells could also present ballooning degeneration with vesicle formation and disruption of dermis [62]. The visualization of cytoplasm eosinophilic inclusion bodies is possible but not common.

The higher virus titres are found in lymphoid tissues ($>10^8$ pfu/g) with lymphoid depletion in the lymph nodes and, in some strains, in the spleen. High loads are also found in secondary cutaneous lesions, the swollen eyelids and particularly in the very swollen tissues at the base of the ears, which are probably important for insect transmission. The viral loads in the lungs or liver are generally lower [59, 60, 63].

This ability to replicate and disseminate *via* lymphocytes, establishing infection at distal sites, is critical to the virulence of the European rabbit [47, 64].

Virus shedding occurs by conjunctival and nasal secretions and by eroded cutaneous lesions. Secondary bacterial infections of the upper respiratory tract and conjunctiva with gram-negative bacteria (e.g., *Pasteurella multocida* and *Bordetella bronchiseptica*) are common, with infection of internal organs less reported [65]. When the duration of the disease is longer (i.e., in infections by less pathogenic strains), pneumonia is a common outcome [42, 66, 67].

MYXV strains can be grouped in five broad virulence grades based on the case fatality rates (CFR), average survival time (AST) and clinical signs [51, 68, 69], ranging from grade 1 to grade 5.

The pathophysiological process of death by myxomatosis is still poorly understood. The key viral proteins involved in the replication and dissemination in *Sylvilagus* species cause local immune suppression in the skin, allowing the virus to persist at this level. In the European rabbit, these proteins cause profound immunosuppression. The virulence of field strains was analysed by infecting small groups of laboratory rabbits, classifying them into five broad grades based on the case fatality rates (CFR), average survival time (AST) and clinical signs [51, 68, 69], namely:

Grade 1: CFR of 99.5%, AST $\leq$ 13 days
Grade 2: CFR of 95–99%, AST 14–16 days
Grade 3A: CFR of 90–95%, AST 17–22 days
Grade 3B: CFR of 70–90%, AST 23–29 days
Grade 4: CFR of 50–70%, AST 29–50 days
Grade 5: CFR less than 50%, AST not determined

Lepus granatensis was considered naturally resistant to myxomatosis, which is endemic in the Iberian Peninsula since 1956 [70]. In 2018, a naturally recombinant myxoma virus (named ha-MYXV or rec-MYXV) emerged in Iberian hare (*L. granatensis*) causing high mortality in the field, representing the first cases of non-sporadic/pathogenic myxomatosis in this species [71, 72]. This recombinant virus has more than 100 small mutations compared to the Lausanne strain, and an insertion of about 2.8 kb disrupting the M009.L gene, the most significant genetic difference, associated with the species barrier jump [72]. This same virus was later found associated with very virulent myxomatosis in domestic and wild rabbits, and the susceptibility of *Oryctolagus cuniculus algirus* to ha-MYXV strains isolated either from Iberian hare or from wild rabbit was also demonstrated [73–76]. More recently, classic MYXV strains were found in Iberian hare (*L. granatensis*) and some cases in co-infection with recombinant MYXV strains [73, 76].

2.1.6 Clinical and laboratorial diagnosis

The clinical diagnosis of the disease is relatively easy although there are no pathognomonic signs and the clinical signs can be confused with other diseases such as Pasteurellosis. The lesions are mainly external and located on the skin, eyelids and genitalia, although respiratory pathology can also be found. The definitive diagnosis is obtained by laboratory techniques that have evolved over the years, namely through isolation in susceptible cell lines, electron microscopy, histopathology (which presents some very suggestive lesions, namely the presence of cytoplasmic inclusion bodies in the cells of the epidermis), among others and, above all, the use of the PCR technique, namely real-time PCR that allows a highly sensitive, specific and quantitative diagnosis in about 3 hours [77]. Recently, a multiplex PCR technique was developed allowing the diagnosis and differentiation the various strains of myxoma virus currently known to be circulating [78].

2.2 *Lagovirus europaeus* (RHDV (GI.1) and RHDV2 (GI.2))

2.2.1 Taxonomic classification

Rabbit haemorrhagic disease virus (RHDV) belongs to *Lagovirus* genus, one of the 11 genera that comprise the *Caliciviridae* family recognized by the International Committee on Taxonomy of Viruses (ICTV) [79]. Genus *Lagovirus* also includes European brown hare syndrome virus (EBHSV) and other non-pathogenic viruses, the rabbit caliciviruses (RCVs) or hare caliciviruses (HCVs) [80].

Rabbit haemorrhagic disease (RHD) can be caused by one of two distinct viruses, namely RHDV, also referred to as RHDVa, *Lagovirus europaeus* GI.1 or simply GI.1, and RHDV2, also known as RHDVb, *Lagovirus europaeus* GI.2 or simply GI.2.

2.2.2 Morphology, genome organization and phylogenetic data

The aetiological agent of rabbit haemorrhagic disease (RHD) is a single-stranded, non-enveloped icosahedral capsid virus with a spherical morphology and a positive-sense RNA [81–83].

The major capsid protein VP1/VP60 forms the structure of the virion and the minor structural protein VP2/VP10 is responsible for stability after the encapsidation of viral RNA, covalently linked to the VPg (viral protein genome-linked), which is essential for replication [80].

The genome is around 7.4 kb (precisely 7437 nucleotides long) to which the 2.2 kb subgenomic RNA (sgRNA) binds to. The genomic RNA is divided into ORF1, encoding a polyprotein that is cleaved into several non-structural proteins and the major structural capsid protein, VP60 (60 kDa), and ORF2 that encodes the minor structural protein called VP10 or VP2 [81, 82, 84].

The viral capsid comprises 90 arch-like dimers of the capsid protein VP60, and 32 cup-shaped depressions, which gives the name to the family *Caliciviridae*, arranged in a T = 3 icosahedral symmetry [85–88]. The electron-dense core has an approximate diameter of 23–25 nm [89, 90].

In the VP60 the main viral antigen, the exposed surface loop—L1 from the P2 subdomain exhibits a higher variability between the strains and contains neutralizing antibody inducing epitopes [91–93]. The cross-protective immunity between the different genotypes is very limited [91–96] and for this reasons, it is predictable that new RHDV genogroups will keep emerging in the future.

2.2.3 Viral replication

The suggested primary site of RHDV replication and entry door (probably by binding to ABH histo-blood group antigens (HBGAs)) is the epithelial cell of the upper respiratory and digestive tracts, being the hepatocyte the major site of replication [97, 98]. The viral genome is released into the cell cytoplasm leading to the direct translation of the viral proteins. In the absence of m7G cap strucures, VPg may play a crucial role in the translation initiation [99, 100] acting as a cap substitute or analogue, interacting with translation initiation factors eIF4E and/or eIF3 [100, 101].

While the translation of ORF1 encoding polyprotein precursor occurs at the initiation codon AUG, the translation of ORF2 encoding VP10 starts by an unusual mechanism of reinitiation after the termination of translation of the preceding major capsid protein VP60 [99]. VP10 can induce hepatocyte apoptosis and virion release and dissemination [102].

2.2.4 Epidemiology (origin, transmission and distribution)

RHDV (*Lagovirus europaeus* GI.1) emerged in Wuxi City, in the last quarter of 1983 in domestic rabbits imported from Germany to the Jiangsu province in China [83, 103], being the first genotype described of rabbit haemorrhagic disease virus (RHDV) [103, 104], that causes a fatal disease in adult rabbits and a subclinical disease in rabbits younger than 4–6 weeks [105, 106]. In the first 12 months after its emergence, the disease killed over 140 million rabbits in China and reached the Europe, namely to Italy, 2 years later [107, 108]. Within 10 years, the disease became endemic in Europe, with severe impact on the European wild rabbit, mainly on the Iberian Peninsula where the specie is a keystone species [14, 23, 109], but also causing sever loses in industrial rabbit farms in both Europe and North Africa [110].

The first cases of RHDV in wild rabbits were reported in Spain in 1988 [111], in Madeira Island (in 1988) and in the Azorean archipelago (Faial Island in 1988, São Jorge Island in 1989 and Santa Maria Island in 1990) (reviewed in Ref. [112]). In the next years, the disease was reported worldwide.

RHDV2 emerged in France in 2010 [113] and quickly replaced the circulating strains of RHDV in most European countries, in the both wild and domestic populations [114–116]. Nowadays, the virus is already reported almost all over the world [112, 113, 117–124].

In the last decade, RHDV2 was reported in several non-habitual species, some representing species barrier jumps including for different mammalian orders, such as small mammals species [96] as well as in Alpine Musk Deer (*Moschus sifanicus*) [125] and Euroasiatic badger (*Melus melus*) [126].

2.2.5 Pathogenesis and disease characterization

RHDV is the etiological agent of the Rabbit Haemorrhagic Disease (RHD), the so-called given the severe dysregulation of the coagulation system.

RHDV integrates the WOAH list of notifiable terrestrial and aquatic animal diseases being a transmissible disease of socio-economic importance within countries, and significant in the international trade of animals and animal products.

The incubation period of RHD induced by RHDV (GI.1) ranges from 1 to 3 days [111, 127] while for RHDV2 (GI.2), it ranges between 3 and 9 days with death occurring 12–36 hours after the onset of fever.

RHDV2 also differs from RHDV in antigenic profile, the apparent lower mortality (5–70%, 20% in average), compared to RHDV [106, 113, 128], age of the animals affected (RHDV2 affects kittens of just 11 days [117]), a longer course of disease of 3–5 days and a higher proportion of rabbits showing subacute-chronic disease comparing with the previous genotypes [106, 113]. The virus has already been detected in leporids other than the European rabbit, namely in the *L. europaeus* [129], *L. capensis* [130], *L. timidus* [131, 132], *L. granatensis* [39], *L. californicus* and *Sylvilagus audubonii* [123].

2.2.6 Clinical and laboratorial diagnosis

The typical (nodular) myxomatosis shows very specific, but not pathognomonic, lesions, particularly nodular thickening of the eyelids, the presence of myxomas and anogenital oedema. The final diagnosis may be achieved by molecular diagnosis according to the WOAH guidelines [133].

Poxviruses can be identified in the skin lesions (myxomas), eyelids and genitalia but also in many other organs attending to the fact that the disease is most often systemic, so in the lungs, liver, spleen and kidney, among others [133]. The diagnosis can be performed through laborious techniques such as the negative-staining electron microscopy (nsEM), histopathology, immunohistochemistry, viral isolation, agar gel immunodiffusion (AGID) and direct immunofluorescence test (dFT) but is currently mostly performed using real-time PCR [78].

2.3 European Brown Hare Syndrome Virus (EBHSV)

2.3.1 Taxonomic classification

Like RHDV, European Brown Hare syndrome Virus (EBHSV) belongs to the *Lagovirus* genus and the *Caliciviridae* family. Although not recognized by the ICTV, the proposed classification [104] for this virus is *Lagovirus europaeus* (species), which includes genogroup GII (EBHSV and hare calicivirus (HaCV)). EBHSV represents the GII.1 genotype that includes three variants (GII.1a, GII.1b and GII.1c).

EBHSV shares with RHDV a phylogenetic relationship, however with distinct antigenic profiles [89, 134].

2.3.2 Epidemiology (origin, transmission and distribution)

The disease was first reported in Gotland island, Sweden, in 1980 and, 1 year later, in the mainland [135]. In the following years, the disease spread to several European countries [136–139] with a huge impact on the wild populations of European Brown hare [140–143].

The European Brown Hare Syndrome (EBHS) shares with RHD many pathophysiological, clinical and epizootic particularities. This disease is also an highly infecto-contagious and fatal disease of the European brown hare (*Lepus europeaus*), the most disseminated hare species, and in lower grade the Mountain hare (*Lepus timidus*) found in the tundra biome [144].

Generally, hares develop an acute form of disease dying a few hours after clinical signals onset. The young hares are also susceptible to infection but due to eventual natural resistance, do not develop disease [89, 144].

EBHSV may be less species-specific than RHD virus and has been recorded as infecting also Eastern cottontails (*S. floridanus*).

2.3.3 Clinical and laboratorial diagnosis

Death is most often the outcome of acute infections, so free-ranging hares may be found dead in the field if not predated. The clinical course is very similar to RHD, with anorexia, depression and neurologic signs secondary to hepatic encephalopathy.

Gross and microscopic lesions may include hepatocellular necrosis, haemorrhages, icterus, inflammatory infiltrates, splenic and/or renal congestion and enlargement [145].

The confirmation of diagnosis may be carried out by molecular techniques namely conventional or real-time PCR as well as using indirect methods that detect antibodies [145].

2.4 Leporid herpesvirus (LeHV-1 to LeHV-5)

2.4.1 Taxonomic classification

Herpesviruses affecting mammals, birds and reptiles belong to *Herpesviridae* family and are highly disseminated in nature, with most animal species have yielded at least one herpesvirus identified [146].

The *Herpesviridae* family includes the subfamilies *Alphaherpesvirinae*, *Betaherpesvirinae* and *Gammaherpesvirinae*. Their members have different biologic properties and distinct classification, supported by phylogenetic data. The *Gammaherpesvirinae* subfamily is divided into four genera, namely *Macavirus*, *Percavirus*, *Lymphocryptovirus* and *Rhadinovirus* [147, 148].

While members of the subfamily *Alphaherpesvirinae* cause rapid lysis in cell culture, members of *Betaherpesvirinae* grow slowly inducing the formation of giant cells in culture, while *Gammaherpesvirinae* typically infect lymphoid tissue, revealing a primary tropism for lymphoid lineage cells [149], which can lead to lymphoproliferative diseases [150] and oncogenesis [151].

At the moment, five herpesviruses were described in Leporids namely the Leporid herpesvirus 1 (LeHV-1), Leporid herpesvirus 2 (LeHV-2), Leporid herpesvirus 3 (LeHV-3), Leporid herpesvirus 4 (LeHV-4) and Leporid herpesvirus 5 (LeHV-5). LeHV-2 and LeHV-3 (reviewed by Refs. [150, 152]) are the most commonly described herpesviruses in rabbits, which alongside LeHV-1 belong to the *Gammaherpesvirinae* subfamily. LeHV-4, an alphaherpesvirus, is the most pathogenic in rabbits, causing fatal infections. Recently, LeHV-5 (Leporid gammaherpesvirus 5) was described affecting the Iberian hare [153].

2.4.2 Morphology and genome organization

The virion structure [146] consists of a core containing a linear dsDNA with 124–295 kb in length, an icosahedral capsid with approximately 125 nm in diameter, one capsomeric structure that serves as the portal for packaging and release of the viral genome, the tegument—an amorphous appearing substance that surrounds the nucleocapsid, and an envelope containing viral glycoprotein spikes on its surface. When mature, the virion size ranges from 120 to 260 nm [154]. The envelope derives from patches of altered nuclear membrane being mainly constituted by viral glycoproteins [155, 156].

The core of a mature virion contains a single dsDNA packed in a torus form [155, 157]. The capsid contains 161 capsomers (10 hexons and 11 pentons), a portal complex with a capsid triangulation (T = 16), preserved in all herpesviruses [158–160]. The non-enveloped capsids could present different forms, namely A (capsids without core), B (capsids containing the assembly scaffold without genome) and C (capsids containing genome without scaffold) [161].

The tegument is a proteinaceous structure between the nucleocapsid and the envelope [146] in general thicker in the virions accumulating in cytoplasmic vacuoles. The tegument proteins closer to the nucleocapsid (inner tegument) are acquired in the nucleus and by interactions with envelope glycoproteins [162] and the subsequent components incorporated in the cytoplasm [162]. The tegument proteins are important in the early phase of infection. The envelope derives from patches of altered nuclear membrane being mainly constituted by viral glycoproteins [155, 156].

The genome of Herpesviridae members encodes between 70 (the smallest) and 200 (the largest) proteins [146].

Herpesvirus genomes can be divided into six groups designated [146] as follows:

a. Exemplified by Human herpesvirus 6 (HHV6), where a large sequence from one terminus is directly repeated at the other terminus;

b. Exemplified by herpesvirus saimiri (SaHV-2), where the terminal sequence is directly repeated numerous times at both termini, with a variable number of repeats at the termini;

c. Exemplified by Epstein-Barr virus (EBV), where the number of direct terminal repeats is smaller and can harbour other direct sequence arrays that subdivide the unique (or quasi unique) sequences of the genome into several well-delineated stretches;

d. Exemplified by Varicella-Zoster virus (VZV), where one terminus is repeated in an inverted orientation internally. The domain consisting of the stretch of unique sequences flanked by inverted repeats (Small or S component) can invert relative to the remaining sequences (Large or L component);

e. Exemplified by herpes simplex virus (HSV) and human cytomegalovirus (HCMV), where the sequences from both termini are repeated in an inverted orientation and juxtaposed internally, dividing the genomes into two components, each of which consists of unique sequences flanked by unrelated pairs of inverted repeats;

f. Exemplified by tupaia herpesvirus 1 (TuHV-1), where the terminal sequences are not identical and are not repeated either directly or in an inverted orientation.

The replication cycle occurs in three major phases: initiation of infection, lytic replication and latency [146]. A biological decision at the cell level is taken to follow either the lytic or the latent pathway, as well, after the initial infection and latency, reactivation of a lytic state [146].

During the lytic replication, a cascade of lytic gene expression occurs, management of the host cell, management of adaptive immune response, replication of virus genome, virus assembly and egress and transmission to other cells and hosts [146]. The restriction of lytic gene expression and expression of latency genes that manage the cell and host defences and maintain the virus genome in the infected cells leads to the latent pathway [146].

2.4.3 Viral replication

The replication cycle is divided into three main phases: initiation of infection, lytic replication and latency [146]. During the initial phase, the binding to the cell receptor occurs, followed by fusion of the viral membrane with the plasma membrane or after endocytosis, management of intrinsic response by tegument proteins, transport of nucleocapsid and tegument-associated IE-activators to the nucleus, injection of viral genome through the nuclear pores and genome chromatinization. The initial interactions with the transcriptional machinery than take place [146]. After these initials steps, the infection triggers a lytic or a latent pathway and in the case of latency, reactivation may occur under certain conditions [146]. During the latent pathway, occurs restriction of lytic gene expression and expression of latency genes that manage the cell and host defences [146].

2.4.4 Epidemiology (origin, transmission and distribution)

The LeHV-5 described in 2020, the only herpesvirus described in hares so far, has been shown to have a great impact on the morbidity and mortality of the Iberian hare, especially when associated with ha-MYXV infections [153]. A survey carried out in Portugal mainland between 2018 and 2021 (Project +Coelho and Project +Coelho 2) showed that approximately 29% of the hares tested (n = 101) were positive for LeHV-5 and all of these were simultaneously coinfected with ha-MYXV.

2.4.5 Pathogenesis and disease characterization

Grossly, vesiculopustular lesions on the eyelids, snout, lips and genitals, necrotizing balanoposthitis and necrosuppurative inflammatory processes on the eyelid and the perivulvar region were observed. Histopathological analysis showed typical herpetic-like vesicles in the epidermis and in the stroma, and a proliferation of pleomorphic spindle cells in the dermis, with nuclei displaying slightly eosinophilic inclusion bodies (Cowdry type A inclusions). The co-infection between LeHV-5 and ha-MYXV leads to an aggressive clinical course and almost invariably to death.

A review of the different herpesviruses and their pathogenies was recently published [153]. Since 2010 no cases of herpesvirus have been reported in both domestic and wild rabbits, and the known herpesviruses have been described very few times over the years.

3. Prevention and disease control of wild leporid viral infections

MYXV grows well in cell lines and live-attenuated viruses through cell passages have been extensively used in Europe as vaccines, due to the inefficacy of inactivated vaccines. On the contrary, until recently, only inactivated vaccines were available [163–168] since RHDV/RHDV2 cannot be grown in cell culture.

The first vaccine available for myxomatosis was an heterologous rabbit fibroma virus [169]. A decade later, an homologous vaccine offering longer immunity was produced based on strains such as MYXV MSD strain, French SG33, MAV, among others, by attenuation in cell culture [170]. Nowadays, these vaccines are still being used and MYXV is also used as a vector for recombinant vaccines harbouring the VP60 of *Lagovirus europaeus*.

Despite the good efficacy of commercial vaccines against myxomatosis, there are still sporadic outbreaks in industrial rabbit farming, with annual rabbit deaths and costs of biosecurity measures [171]. The outbreaks in industrial rabbit farming often result from vaccine failures not associated with the vaccine itself, but rather with the route of administration, as it has been demonstrated that the intradermal route triggers a better seroconversion than other routes, namely the subcutaneous route, the most commonly used [172]. This fact exemplifies the need and benefits of bringing the productive sector closer to the scientific researchers in order to standardize more effective methods of administration and control of this and other diseases. In fact, the recently emerging ha-MYXV, which has been shown to infect wild and domestic rabbits as well, is highly pathogenic, but commercial vaccine strains have been shown to be effective in preventing disease in rabbits [73–75].

On the other hand, the low applicability of vaccination in the wild hampers a practical solution to contain the virus, resulting in the continuous source of infection and circulation of the virus. Myxomatosis has had a major impact on wild rabbit and Iberian hare populations since its emergence leading to abrupt reductions and local extinctions [3, 173–176] with a chain effect, especially in the Mediterranean ecosystems, due to the role of keystone species in food chains [5].

Myxomatosis treatment is possible, but merely symptomatic, considering that there are no antivirals tested for this disease, being a utopia in the case of wild species due to the difficulty in capture and administration. Moreover, treatment is not recommended, due to the risk of environmental contamination and transmission potentiation during treatment (taking into account the dispersion by biting insects and mechanical transmission), and the possibility of the animals becoming carriers [177]. For this reason, the only current way of controlling the disease is through vaccination and biosecurity measures, which can be adapted, partially, to the wild.

Since 2018, thousands of hares died in Portugal and Spain in the field due to ha-MYXV, causing a reduction of more than 50% in the wild populations of both countries, which will lead to the attribution of Vulnerable status by the IUCN in late 2022. The long-term impact of this new recombinant virus on the Iberian hare and the wild rabbit is yet to be known. However, the possibilities available for the recovery of both species are predictably low, especially for the Iberian hare, which has a dynamic reproduction much lower than the wild rabbit.

4. Conclusions

In recent years, the wild rabbit and the Iberian hare have been gaining growing interest from the academy, civil society, the environmental and ecological organizations and policy makers. A clear example of these was the Projects +Coelho, implemented following the constitution of a working group by Dispatch no. 4757/2017 of 31 May of the Portuguese Ministry of Agriculture, to respond to the effect of rabbit haemorrhagic disease in the rabbit population, the Mixo*lepus* project in Spain in response to the emergence of ha-MYXV or the recently approved LIFE Iberconejo with an allocation of around 2 million euros for 3 years. These, and other investments, are fully justified given the importance of the wild rabbit in the Mediterranean ecosystem, where its role is so decisive that some ecologists call the Iberian Peninsula the "rabbit's ecosystem" [5]. In fact, the most paradigmatic conservation projects in the Iberian Peninsula take place on areas with rabbit abundance namely the projects involving Iberian lynx (Life+IBERLINCE), Black vulture (Parque Natural do Tejo Internacional) and Imperial eagle (Parque Natural do Vale do Guadiana and ZPE of Castro Verde), among others.

Viral diseases have been identified as the main causes of the leporid decline [115, 116]. The importance and severity of viruses were evidenced during the 3 years of field work performed within the scope of this doctoral thesis when it was possible to testify the emergence of myxomatosis in Iberian hare by the natural recombinant ha-MYXV [71], cases of co-infection with ha-MYXV and classic MYXV in hares and rabbits, never detected before [76], co-infection with MYXV and RHDV2 [178] the spillover of the ha-MYXV (natural recombinant myxoma virus) from hares to rabbits [74, 75], the identification of a herpesvirus in hares undergoing myxomatosis [74, 75] not described before and the detection of an Iberian hare infected with rabbit haemorrhagic disease [39]. During the health analysis of wild rabbit cadavers found in mainland Portugal between 2018 and 2020, MYXV was found in about 27.81% of the animals [3]. Also in the scope of the virological analyses of leporid cadavers found in mainland Portugal between 2018 and 2020, RHDV2 was found in about 48.52% of the rabbits and 84.21% of the hares [3]. During the health analysis of rabbit cadavers found in mainland Portugal between 2018 and 2020, RHDV2 and MYXV were detected in 76.33% [116] and associated with animal death.

5. Future perspectives

Currently, only the viral infections described above are associated with a major impact on wild leporid populations, with particular relevance to myxoma viruses and Lagoviruses. However, because only what is sought is found, we cannot guarantee that other viruses are not affecting the wild populations. In fact, beside a few time-limited studies, no robust and long-term sanitary surveillances and research programmes have been conducted in wild leporid species. It is therefore crucial to invest in continuous monitoring of these species, that are essential for ecosystems, with a special focus on the Mediterranean basin.

The Iberian hare is an endemic specie of the Iberian Peninsula whose populations are considered stable by the IUCN holding a 'least concern' conservation status [179]. However, its status will be likely reviewed this year, probably to Vulnerable, given the trends registered after 2018. If the current downward trend in the field continues, and if myxomatosis also becomes endemic in this species, the *L. granatensis* conservation status will be progressively worsened to the point of functional extinction of a species that is iconic for the Iberian Peninsula.

The progressive loss, fragmentation and changes in habitat and wildlife management are putting leporids, and other species around the world, at great risk. Only a professional and integrated management of these species will allow them to remain as key species in our ecosystems. Otherwise we will continue to observe the drastic cascading effects of leporid decrease on other species.

According to the World Wildlife Fund (WWF) 'Living Planet 2020' report, global wildlife populations have declined by an average of 60% over the past 40 years; therefore, it is urgent to adopt practical measures of positive impact in short and medium terms [180].

Today, we have the knowledge and the means to develop solutions, often retained by lack of political will and social and ecological motivation, to make pioneering and innovative decisions that will allow paradigm shifts. One such example is the use of new microbiological solutions, namely recombinant vaccines, transgenic foods that express immunizing proteins, the use of artificial intelligence and machine learning to deliver molecules. All these resources, and many more, are now a reality, but they still need to be implemented in wildlife.

Acknowledgements

The authors thank the Virology laboratory technical staff of the National Institute for Agricultural and Veterinary Research (INIAV, I.P.). Some data reported here resulted from funding by Fundo Florestal Permanente (Government of Portugal) within the scope of the Action Plan for the Control of Rabbit Viral Haemorrhagic Disease (Project +COELHO, Dispatch no. 4757/2017 of 31 May), Fundação para a Ciência e Tecnologia (FCT, UIDB/00276/2020), Lisbon, Portugal and the Interdisciplinary Research Centre on Animal Health (CIISA), Faculty of Veterinary Medicine, University of Lisbon, Portugal.

Conflict of interest

The authors declare no conflict of interest.

Author details

Fábio A. Abade dos Santos[1,2,3,4*], Teresa Fagulha[1], Sílvia S. Barros[1], Margarida Henriques[1], Ana Duarte[1], Fernanda Ramos[1], Tiago Luís[1] and Margarida D. Duarte[1,2,3]

1 National Institute of Agrarian and Veterinarian Research, Oeiras, Portugal

2 Centre for Interdisciplinary Research in Animal Health (CIISA), Faculdade de Medicina Veterinária, Universidade de Lisboa, Avenida da Universidade Técnica, Lisbon, Portugal

3 Associate Laboratory for Animal and Veterinary Sciences (AL4AnimalS), Lisbon, Portugal

4 Faculdade de Medicina Veterinária, Universidade Lusófona de Humanidades e Tecnologia, Lisboa, Portugal

*Address all correspondence to: fabio.abade@iniav.pt

References

[1] Asher RJ, Meng J, Wible JR, McKenna MC, Rougier GW, Dashzeveg D, et al. Stem Lagomorpha and the antiquity of Glires. Science. 2005;**307**(5712):1091-1094

[2] Alves P, Ferrand N, Hackländer K. Lagomorph Biology: Evolution, Ecology, and Conservation. XVIII. Zoology, Animal Migration, Evolutionary Theory. Heidelber: Springer; 2008

[3] Duarte MD, Carvalho CL, dos Santos FA, Monteiro J, Monteiro M, Carvalho PM, et al. The health and future of the six hare species in Europe: A closer look at the Iberian hare. In: Argente M-J, de la Luz García Pardo M, Dalton KP, editors. Lagomorpha Characteristics. Rijeka: IntechOpen; 2021. pp. 1-34. Available from: https://doi.org/10.5772/intechopen.91876

[4] Long J. Introduced Mammals of the World. Their History, Distribution and Influence. Victoria, Australia: CSIRO Publishing; 2003. p. 612. Available from: https://ebooks.publish.csiro.au/content/9780643090156/9780643090156

[5] Delibes-Mateos M, Delibes M, Ferreras P, Villafuerte R. Key role of European rabbits in the conservation of the western Mediterranean Basin hotspot. Conservation Biology. 2008;**22**(5):1106-1117

[6] Wilson D, Lacher T, Mittermeier R. Lagomorphs and rodents I. In: Handbook of the Mammals of the World. Vol. 6. Barcelona, Spain: Lynx Edicions; 2016

[7] Palden B, Smith A, Senko J, Siladan M. Plateau Pika *Ochotona curzoniae* poisoning campaign reduces carnivore abundance in Southern Qinghai, China. Mammal Study. 2016;**41**:1-8

[8] Tablado Z, Revilla E, Palomares F. Breeding like rabbits: Global patterns of variability and determinants of European wild rabbit reproduction. Ecography. 2009;**32**(2):310-320

[9] Vaughan T, Ryan J, Czaplewski N. Mammalogy. Sudbury, Mass.: Jones and Bartlett Publishers; 2011

[10] Gómez Sal A, Rey Benayas JM, López-Pintor A, Rebollo S. Role of disturbance in maintaining a savanna-like pattern in Mediterranean *Retama sphaerocarpa* shrubland. Journal of Vegetation Science. 1999;**10**:365-370

[11] Kuijper DPJ, Nijhoff DJ, Bakker JP. Herbivory and competition slow down invasion of a tall grass along a productivity gradient. Oecologia. 2004;**141**(3):452-459. Available from: https://edepot.wur.nl/45059

[12] Kuijper DPJ, Beek P, van Wieren SE, Bakker JP. Time-scale effects in the interaction between a large and a small herbivore. Basic and Applied Ecology. 2008;**9**(2):126-134. Available from: https://www.sciencedirect.com/science/article/pii/S1439179106001204

[13] Gálvez-Bravo L, López-Pintor A, Rebollo S, Gómez-Sal A. European rabbit (*Oryctolagus cuniculus*) engineering effects promote plant heterogeneity in Mediterranean dehesa pastures. Journal of Arid Environments. 2011;**75**(9):779-786. Available from: https://www.sciencedirect.com/science/article/pii/S0140196311001029

[14] Delibes-Mateos M, Redpath SM, Angulo E, Ferreras P, Villafuerte R. Rabbits as a keystone species in southern Europe. Biological Conservation. 2007;**137**(1):149-156

[15] Delibes M, Hiraldo F. The rabbit as a prey in the Iberian Mediterranean ecossystem. In: Myers K, MacInnes CD, editors. Proceedings of the World Lagomorph Conference (1979). Ontario: University of Guelph; 1981. pp. 654-663

[16] John EF, Sharples CM, Bell DJ. Habitat correlates of European rabbit (*Oryctolagus cuniculus*) distribution after the spread of RVHD in Cadiz Province, Spain. Journal of Zoology. 1999;**249**(01):83-96. Available from: http://dx.doi.org/10.1017/S0952836999009085

[17] Ferrer M, Negro JJ. The near extinction of two large European predators: Super specialists pay a price. Conservation Biology. 2004;**18**(2):344-349. Available from: http://www.jstor.org/stable/3589211 [Cited: 24 September 2022]

[18] Anticona SJ, Olmos EF, Parent JR, Rutti DM, Velasco BA, Hoese W. Greater roadrunner (*Geococcyx californianus*) kills juvenile desert cottontail (*Sylvilagus audubonii*). The Free Library; 01 March 2013. Available from: https://www.thefreelibrary.com/Greater roadrunner (*Geococcyx californianus*) kills juvenile desert...-a0324981091 [Cited: 24 September 2022]

[19] O'Donoghue M. Early survival of juvenile snowshoe hares. Ecology. 1994;**75**(6):1582-1592. Available from: https://esajournals.onlinelibrary.wiley.com/doi/abs/10.2307/1939619

[20] Palomares F, Gaona P, Ferreras P, Delibes M. Positive effects on game species of top predators by controlling smaller predator populations: An example with lynx, mongooses, and rabbits. Conservation Biology. 1995;**9**(2):295-305. Available from: http://www.jstor.org/stable/2386774 [Cited: 24 September 2022]

[21] Cowling RM, Rundel PW, Lamont BB, Arroyo MK, Arianoutsou M. Plant diversity in Mediterranean-climate regions. Trees. 1996;**11**(9):362-366

[22] Médail F, Quézel P. Biodiversity hotspots in the mediterranean basin: Setting global conservation priorities. Conservation Biology. 1999;**13**(6):1510-1513

[23] Villafuerte R, Calvete C, Blanco JC, Lucientes J. Incidence of viral hemorrhagic disease in wild rabbit populations in Spain. Mammalia. 1995;**59**(4):651-660

[24] Bell DJ, Webb NJ. Effects of climate on reproduction in the European wild rabbit (*Oryctolagus cuniculus*). Journal of Zoology. 1991;**224**:639-648

[25] Calvete C. Modeling the effect of population dynamics on the impact of rabbit hemorrhagic disease. Conservation Biology. 2006;**20**(4):1232-1241

[26] Lowe S, Browne M, Boudjelas S, De Poorter M. 100 of the World's Worst Invasive Alien Species A selection from the Global Invasive Species Database. Published by The Invasive Species Specialist Group (ISSG) a specialist group of the Species Survival Commission (SSC) of the World Conservation Union (IUCN). First published as special lift-out in Aliens 12, December 2000. p. 12. Updated and reprinted version: November 2004

[27] Pimentel D, McNair S, Janecka J, Wightman J, Simmonds C, O'Connell C, et al. Economic and environmental threats of alien plant, animal, and microbe invasions. Agriculture, Ecosystems and Environment. 2001;**84**(1):1-20

[28] Soriguer RC. El conejo, *Oryctolagus cuniculus* (L), en Andalucía Occidental: Parámetos corporales y curva de crecimiento. Acta Vertebr. 1980;**7**(1):83-90

[29] Chapman JA, Flux J. Rabbits, Hares and Pikas: Status Survey and

Conservation Action Plan. Gland, Switzerland: IUCN; 1990

[30] von Holst D, Hutzelmeyer H, Kaetzke P, Khaschei M, Rödel HG, Schrutka H. Social rank, fecundity and lifetime reproductive success in wild European rabbits (*Oryctolagus cuniculus*). Behavioral Ecology and Sociobiology. 2002;**51**:245-254

[31] Flux JE. Timing of the breeding season in the hare, *Lepus europaeus* Pallas, and rabbit, *Oryctolagus cuniculus* (L.). Mammalia. 1965;**29**:557-562

[32] Fontanesi L, Di Palma F, Flicek P, Smith AT, Thulin CG, Alves PC, et al. LaGomiCs—Lagomorph genomics consortium: An international collaborative effort for sequencing the genomes of an entire mammalian order. The Journal of Heredity. 2016;**107**(4):295-308

[33] Fuentes MV, Coello JR, Bargues M, Valero M, Esteban J, Fons R, et al. Small mammals (Lagomorpha and Rodentia) and fascioliasis transmission in the Northern Bolivian Altiplano endemic zone. Research and Reviews in Parasitology. 1997;**57**:115-121

[34] Kleiman F, González N, Rubel D, Wisniveksy C. *Fasciola hepatica* (Linnaeus, 1758) (Trematoda, Digenea) en liebres europeas (*Lepus europaeus*, Pallas 1778) (Lagomorpha, Leporidae) en la región Cordillerana Patagónica, Chubut, Argentina. Parasitología latinoamericana. 2004;**59**(1-2):68-71

[35] Tiawsirisup S, Platt KB, Tucker BJ, Rowley WA. Eastern cottontail rabbits (*Sylvilagus floridanus*) develop West Nile virus viremias sufficient for infecting select mosquito species. Vector Borne and Zoonotic Diseases. 2005;**5**(4):342-350

[36] Gallo MG, Tizzani P, Peano A, Rambozzi L, Meneguz PG. Eastern cottontail (*Sylvilagus floridanus*) as carrier of dermatophyte fungi. Mycopathologia. 2005;**160**(2):163-166

[37] Paolo T, Stefano C, Rossi L, Padraig D, Giuseppe MP. Invasive species and their parasites: Eastern cottontail rabbit Sylvilagus floridanus and Trichostrongylus affinis (Graybill, 1924) from Northwestern Italy. Parasitology Research; 2014. p. 113. DOI: 10.1007/s00436-014-3768-1

[38] Abade dos Santos FA, Portela SJ, Nogueira T, Carvalho CL, de Sousa R, Duarte MD. Harmless or threatening? Interpreting the results of molecular diagnosis in the context of virus-host relationships. Frontiers in Microbiology. 2021;**12**:1-8. Available from: https://www.frontiersin.org/article/10.3389/fmicb.2021.647730

[39] Velarde R, Abrantes J, Lopes AM, Estruch J, Côrte-Real JV, Esteves PJ, et al. Spillover event of recombinant *Lagovirus europaeus*/GI.2 into the Iberian hare (*Lepus granatensis*) in Spain. Transboundary and Emerging Diseases. 2021;**68**(6):3187-3193

[40] Zhou J, Sun W, Wang J, Guo J, Yin W, Wu N, et al. Characterization of the H5N1 highly pathogenic avian influenza virus derived from wild pikas in China. Journal of Virology. 2009;**83**(17):8957-8964

[41] Zhu W, Yang J, Lu S, Jin D, Wu S, Pu J, et al. Discovery and evolution of a divergent coronavirus in the plateau pika from China that extends the host range of alphacoronaviruses. Frontiers in Microbiology. 2021;**12**:755599

[42] Kerr PJ, Liu J, Cattadori I, Ghedin E, Read AF, Holmes EC. Myxoma virus and the leporipoxviruses: An evolutionary paradigm. Viruses. 2015;7(3):1020-1061

[43] Morales M, Ramírez MA, Cano MJ, Párraga M, Castilla J, Pérez-Ordoyo LI,

et al. Genome comparison of a nonpathogenic myxoma virus field strain with its ancestor, the virulent Lausanne strain. Journal of Virology. 2009;**83**(5):2397-2403

[44] Cameron C, Hota-Mitchell S, Chen L, Barrett J, Cao JX, Macaulay C, et al. The complete dna sequence of myxoma virus. Virology. 1999;**264**(2):298-318

[45] Kerr P, McFadden G. Immune responses to myxoma virus. Viral Immunology. 2002;**15**(2):229-246

[46] Upton C, Slack S, Hunter AL, Ehlers A, Roper RL. Poxvirus orthologous clusters: Toward defining the minimum essential poxvirus genome. Journal of Virology. 2003;**77**(13):7590-7600

[47] Kerr PJ. Myxomatosis in Australia and Europe: A model for emerging infectious diseases. Antiviral Research. 2012;**93**(3):387-415. Available from: http://dx.doi.org/10.1016/j.antiviral.2012.01.009

[48] McFadden G. Poxvirus tropism. Nature Reviews Microbiology. Mar 2005;**3**(3):201-213. DOI: 10.1038/nrmicro1099. PMID: 15738948; PMCID: PMC4382915

[49] Moss B. Poxviridae. In: Knipe DM, Howley PM, editor. Fields Virology. Vol. 2. 6th ed. Philadelphia: Lippincott Williams & Wilkins; 2013. pp. 2129-2159

[50] Broyles SS. Vaccinia virus transcription. Journal of General Virology. Sep 2003;**84**(Pt 9):2293-2303. DOI: 10.1099/vir.0.18942-0. PMID: 12917449

[51] Fenner F, Ratcliffe FN. Myxomatosis. London, UK: Cambridge University Press; 1965

[52] Barlow A, Lawrence K, Everest D, Dastjerdi A, Finnegan C, Steinbach F. Confirmation of myxomatosis in a European brown hare in Great Britain. The Veterinary Record. 2014;**175**(3):75-76

[53] Wibbelt G, Frölich K. Infectious Diseases in European Brown Hare (Lepus europaeus). Wildlife Biology in Practice. 2005;**1**(1):86-93. DOI: 10.2461/wbp.2005.1.11

[54] Sanarelli G. Das myxomatogene virus. Beitrag zum Studer Krankheitserreger ausserhalb des sichtbaren. Cent f Bakt. 1898;**1**(23):865

[55] Arentsen P. Control biológico del conejo: difusión del virus mixomatosis cuniculus, por contagio directo, en la Isla Grande de Tierra del Fuego. Boletín Ganad (Punta Arenas). 1954;**43**:1-26

[56] Kerr PJ, Best SM. Myxoma virus in rabbits myxoma virus and myxomatosis biological control for the myxomatosis in rabbits in Australia: Development of resistance associated with. Revue Scientifique et Technique. 1998;**7**(1):256-268

[57] Saint KM, French N, Kerr P. Genetic variation in Australian isolates of myxoma virus: An evolutionary and epidemiological study. Archives of Virology. 2001;**146**(6):1105-1123

[58] Alves JM, Carneiro M, Cheng JY, de Matos AL, Rahman MM, Loog L, et al. Parallel adaptation of rabbit populations to myxoma virus. Science (80-.). 2019;**363**(6433):1319-1326. Available from: https://www.science.org/doi/abs/10.1126/science.aau7285

[59] Fenner F, Woodroofe GM. The pathogenesis of infectious myxomatosis; the mechanism of infection and the immunological response in the European rabbit (*Oryctolagus cuniculus*). British Journal of Experimental Pathology. 1953;**34**(4):400-411

[60] Best SM, Kerr PJ. Coevolution of host and virus: The pathogenesis of virulent and attenuated strains of myxoma virus in resistant and susceptible European rabbits. Virology. 2000;**267**(1):36-48

[61] Best SM, Collins SV, Kerr PJ. Coevolution of host and virus: Cellular localization of virus in myxoma virus infection of resistant and susceptible European rabbits. Virology. 2000;**277**(1):76-91

[62] Kerr PJ, Cattadori IM, Sim D, Liu J, Holmes EC, Read AF. Divergent evolutionary pathways of myxoma virus in Australia: Virulence phenotypes in susceptible and partially resistant rabbits indicate possible selection for transmissibility. Journal of Virology. 2022;**96**(20):e00886-e00822

[63] Hurst EW. Myxoma and the Shope fibroma. I. The histology of myxoma. British Journal of Experimental Pathology. 1937;**18**:1-15

[64] Spiesschaert B, Mcfadden G, Hermans K, Nauwynck H, Van De Walle GR. The current status and future directions of myxoma virus, a master in immune evasion. Veterinary Research. 2011;**42**(1):76. Available from: http://www.veterinaryresearch.org/content/42/1/76

[65] Hobbs J. Studies of the nature of infectious myxoma of rabbits. American Journal of Hygiene. 1928;**8**:800-839

[66] Marlier D, Mainil J, Sulon J, Beckers JF, Linden A, Vindevogel H. Study of the virulence of five strains of amyxomatous myxoma virus in crossbred New Zealand white/Californian conventional rabbits, with evidence of long-term testicular infection in recovered animals. Journal of Comparative Pathology. 2000;**122**(2-3):101-113

[67] Duclos P, Tuaillon P, Joubert L. Histopathologie de l' atteinte cutanéo-muqueuse et pulmonaire de la myxomatose. Bulletin de l'Academie Veterinaire. 1983;**56**:95-104

[68] Fenner BYF, Marshall ID. A comparison of the virulence for european rabbits (*Oryctolagus cuniculus*) of strains of myxoma virus recovered in the field in Australia, Europe and America. Journal of Hygiene. 1957;**55**(2):149-191

[69] Fenner F, Woodroofe GM. Changes in the virulence and antigenic structure of strains of myxoma virus recovered from Australian wild rabbits between 1950 and 1964. The Australian Journal of Experimental Biology and Medical Science. 1965;**43**:359-370

[70] Fenner F, Fantini B. History of myxomatosis—An experiment in evolution. In: Biological Control of Vertebrate Pests. New York, USA: CABI Publishing, Oxford; 1999

[71] Carvalho CL, Abade Dos Santos FA, Monteiro M, Carvalho P, Mendonça P, Duarte MD. First cases of myxomatosis in Iberian hares (*Lepus granatensis*) in Portugal. Veterinary Record Case Reports. 2020;**8**(2):1-5. Available from: https://vetrecordcasereports.bmj.com/content/8/2/e001044

[72] Dalton KP, Martín JM, Nicieza I, Podadera A, Llano D, Casais R, et al. Myxoma virus jumps species to the Iberian hare. Transboundary and Emerging Diseases. 2019;**66**(6):2218-2226. Available from: https://onlinelibrary.wiley.com/doi/abs/10.1111/tbed.13296

[73] Abade dos Santos FA, Carvalho CL, Valente PCLG, Armés H, Reemers SS, Peleteiro MC, et al. Evaluation of commercial myxomatosis vaccines against recombinant myxoma virus (ha-MYXV) in Iberian hare and wild rabbit. Vaccine. 2022;**10**(3):356. Available from: https://www.mdpi.com/2076-393X/10/3/356

[74] Abade dos Santos F, Carvalho C, Monteiro M, Carvalho P, Mendonça P, Peleteiro MC, et al. Recombinant myxoma virus infection associated with high mortality in rabbit farming (*Oryctolagus cuniculus*). Transboundary and Emerging Diseases. 2020;**68**(4):2616-2621

[75] Abade dos Santos F, Carvalho C, Pinto A, Rai R, Monteiro M, Carvalho P, et al. Detection of recombinant hare myxoma virus in wild rabbits (*Oryctolagus cuniculus* algirus). Viruses. 2020;**12**(1127):1-12

[76] Abade dos Santos FA, Dalton KP, Casero M, Álvarez ÁL, Parra F, Carvalho CL, et al. Co-infection by classic MYXV and ha-MYXV in Iberian hare (*Lepus granatensis*) and European wild rabbit (*Oryctolagus cuniculus* algirus). Transboundary and Emerging Diseases. 2022;**69**(4):1684-1690

[77] Duarte MD, Barros SC, Henriques AM, Fagulha MT, Ramos F, Luís T, et al. Development and validation of a real time PCR for the detection of myxoma virus based on the diploid gene M000.5L/R. Journal of Virological Methods. 2013;**196**:219-224. Available from: http://dx.doi.org/10.1016/j.jviromet.2013.11.014

[78] Abade dos Santos FA, Carvalho CL, Parra F, Dalton KP, Peleteiro MC. A quadruplex qPCR for detection and differentiation of classic and natural recombinant myxoma virus strains of leporids. International Journal of Molecular Sciences. 2021;**22**(21):12052

[79] Vinjé J, Estes MK, Esteves P, Green KY, Katayama K, Knowles NJ, et al. ICTV virus taxonomy profile: Caliciviridae. The Journal of General Virology. 2019;**100**(11):1469-1470. Available from: https://www.microbiologyresearch.org/content/journal/jgv/10.1099/jgv.0.001332

[80] ICTV IC on T of V. Genus: Lagovirus [Internet]. 2021. Available from: https://talk.ictvonline.org/ictvreports/ictv_online_report/positive-sense-rna-viruses/w/caliciviridae/1163/genus-lagovirus [Cited: 10 January 2021]

[81] Meyers G, Wirblich C, Thiel HJ. Rabbit hemorrhagic disease virus-molecular cloning and nucleotide sequencing of a calicivirus genome. Virology. 1991;**184**(2):664-676

[82] Ohlinger VF, Haas B, Meyers G, Weiland F, Thiel H-J. Identification and characterization of the virus causing rabbit hemorrhagic disease. Journal of Virology. 1990;**64**(7):3331-3336

[83] Parra F, Prieto M. Purification and characterization of a calicivirus as the causative agent of a lethal hemorrhagic disease in rabbits. Journal of Virology. 1990;**64**(8):4013-4015

[84] Wirblich C, Thiel HJ, Meyers G. Genetic map of the calicivirus rabbit hemorrhagic disease virus as deduced from in vitro translation studies. Journal of Virology. 1996;**70**(11):7974-7983. Available from: http://jvi.asm.org/content/70/11/7974.short

[85] Bárcena J, Verdaguer N, Roca R, Morales M, Angulo I, Risco C, et al. The coat protein of rabbit hemorrhagic disease virus contains a molecular switch at the N-terminal region facing the inner surface of the capsid. Virology. 2004;**322**(1):118-134

[86] Luque D, Gonzalez JM, Gomez-Blanco J, Marabini R, Chichon J, Mena I, et al. Epitope insertion at the N-terminal molecular switch of the rabbit hemorrhagic disease virus T=3 capsid protein leads to larger T=4 capsids. Journal of Virology. 2012;**86**(12):6470-6480. Available from: http://jvi.asm.org/cgi/doi/10.1128/JVI.07050-11

[87] Valicek L, Smid B, Rodak L, Kudrna J. Electron and immunoelectron

microscopy of rabbit haemorrhagic disease virus (RHDV). Archives of Virology. 1990;**112**:71-275

[88] Thouvenin E, Laurent S, Madelaine MF, Rasschaert D, Vautherot JF, Hewat EA. Bivalent binding of a neutralising antibody to a calicivirus involves the torsional flexibility of the antibody hinge. Journal of Molecular Biology. 1997;**270**(2):238-246. Available from: http://www.ncbi.nlm.nih.gov/pubmed/9236125

[89] Capucci L, Scicluna M, Lavazza A. Diagnosis of viral haemorrhagic disease of rabbits and the European brown hare syndrome. Revue Scientifique et Technique. 1991;**10**:347-370

[90] Sibilia M, Boniotti MB, Angoscini P, Capucci L, Rossi C. Two independent pathways of expression lead to self-assembly of the rabbit hemorrhagic disease virus capsid protein. Journal of Virology. 1995;**69**(9):5812-5815. Available from: http://www.pubmedcentral.nih.gov/articlerender.fcgi?artid=189447&tool=pmcentrez&rendertype=abstract

[91] Capucci L, Frigoli G, Ronshold L, Lavazza A, Brocchi E, Rossi C. Antigenicity of the rabbit hemorrhagic disease virus studied by its reactivity with monoclonal antibodies Lorenzo. Virus Research. 1995;**37**:221-238

[92] Capucci L, Fallacara F, Grazioli S, Lavazza A, Pacciarini ML, Brocchi E. A further step in the evolution of rabbit hemorrhagic disease virus: The appearance of the first consistent antigenic variant. Virus Research. 1998;**58**(1-2):115-126

[93] Schirrmeier H, Reimann I, Granzow H, Riems I. Pathogenic, antigenic and molecular properties of rabbit haemorrhagic disease virus (RHDV) isolated from vaccinated rabbits: Detection and characterization of antigenic variants. Archives of Virology. 1999;**144**(4):719-735

[94] Kinnear M, Linde CC. Capsid gene divergence in rabbit hemorrhagic disease virus. The Journal of General Virology. 2010;**91**(1):174-181

[95] Dalton KP, Nicieza I, Abrantes J, Esteves PJ, Parra F. Spread of new variant RHDV in domestic rabbits on the Iberian peninsula. Veterinary Microbiology. 2014;**169**(1-2):67-73

[96] Calvete C, Mendoza M, Sarto M, Jiménez de Bagués MP, Luján L, Molín J, et al. Detection of rabbit hemorrhagic disease virus GI. 2/RHDV2/B in the mediterranean pine vole (*Microtus duodecimcostatus*) and white-toothed shrew (*Crocidura russula*). Journal of Wildlife Diseases. 2019;**55**(2):467-472

[97] Guillon P, Ruvoën-Clouet N, Le Moullac-Vaidye B, Marchandeau S, Le Pendu J. Association between expression of the H histo-blood group antigen, α1,2fucosyltransferases polymorphism of wild rabbits, and sensitivity to rabbit hemorrhagic disease virus. Glycobiology. 2009;**19**(1):21-28

[98] Ruvoën-Clouet N, Ganiere JP, Andre-Fontaine G, Blanchard D, Le Pendu J. Binding of rabbit hemorrhagic disease virus to antigens of the ABH histo-blood group family. Journal of Virology. 2000;**74**(24):11950-11954. Available from: http://www.pubmedcentral.nih.gov/articlerender.fcgi?artid=112478&tool=pmcentrez&rendertype=abstract

[99] Meyers G. Translation of the minor capsid protein of a calicivirus is initiated by a novel termination-dependent reinitiation mechanism. The Journal of Biological Chemistry. 2003;**278**(36):34051-34060

[100] Daughenbaugh KF, Fraser CS, Hershey JWB, Hardy ME.

The genome-linked protein VPg of the Norwalk virus binds eIF3, suggesting its role in translation initiation complex recruitment. The EMBO Journal. 2003;**22**(11):2852-2859

[101] Goodfellow I, Chaudhry Y, Gioldasi I, Gerondopoulos A, Natoni A, Labrie L, et al. Calicivirus translation initiation requires an interaction between VPg and eIF4E. EMBO Reports. 2005;**6**(10):968-972. Available from: http://embor.embopress.org/cgi/doi/10.1038/sj.embor.7400510

[102] Liu G, Ni Z, Yun T, Yu B, Chen L, Zhao W, et al. A DNA-launched reverse genetics system for rabbit hemorrhagic disease virus reveals that the VP2 protein is not essential for virus infectivity. The Journal of General Virology. 2008;**89**(12):3080-3085

[103] Liu S, Xue H, Pu B, Qian N. A new viral disease in rabbit. Animal Husbandry and Veterinary Medicine. 1984;**16**:253-255

[104] Le Pendu J, Abrantes J, Bertagnoli S, Guitton J-S, Le Gall-Reculé G, Lopes AM, et al. Proposal for a unified classification system and nomenclature of lagoviruses. The Journal of General Virology. 2017;**98**(7):1658-1666. Available from: https://doi.org/10.1099/jgv.0.000840

[105] Chasey D. Rabbit haemorrhagic disease: The new scourge of *Oryctolagus cuniculus*. Laboratory Animals. 1997;**31**(1):33-44

[106] Office International des Epizooties. OIE Rabbit Haemorrhagic Disease. In: OIE Terrestrial Manual 2018. Paris, France: Office International des Epizooties; 2018. pp. 1389-1406. Available online: www.oie.int

[107] Xu W. Viral haemorrhagic disease of rabbits in the People's Republic of China: Epidemiology and virus characterisation. Revue Scientifique et Technique. 1991;**10**:393-408

[108] Rouco C, Aguayo-adán JA, Santoro S, Abrantes J, Delibes-mateos M. Worldwide rapid spread of the novel rabbit haemorrhagic disease virus (GI.2/RHDV2/b). Transboundary and Emerging Diseases. 2019;**66**(4):1762-1764

[109] Argüello J, Llanos A, Pérez L. Enfermedad hemorrágica del conejo en España. MedVet. 1988;**5**:645-650 [in Spanish]

[110] Morisse J, Le Gall G, Boilletot E. Hepatitis of viral origin in Leporidae: Introduction and aetiological hypotheses. Revue Scientifique et Technique. 1991;**10**:283-295

[111] Arguello-Villares JL, Llanos Pellitero A, Perez Ordoyo Garcia LM. Enfermedad vírica hemorrágica del conejo en Espana. Medicina Veterinaria. 1988;**5**:645-650

[112] Duarte M, Carvalho C, Bernardo S, Barros S, Benevides S, Flor L, et al. Rabbit haemorrhagic disease virus 2 (RHDV2) outbreak in Azores: Disclosure of common genetic markers and phylogenetic segregation within the European strains. Infection, Genetics and Evolution. 2015;**35**:163-171. Available from: http://dx.doi.org/10.1016/j.meegid.2015.08.005

[113] Le Gall-Reculé G, Lavazza A, Marchandeau S, Bertagnoli S, Zwingelstein F, Cavadini P, et al. Emergence of a new lagovirus related to rabbit haemorrhagic disease virus. Veterinary Research. 2013;**44**(1):1-13

[114] Calvete C, Sarto P, Calvo AJ, Monroy F, Calvo JH. Could the new rabbit haemorrhagic disease virus variant (RHDVb) be fully replacing classical

RHD strains in the Iberian Peninsula? World Rabbit Science. 2014;**22**:91-91

[115] Duarte MD, Carvalho CL, Abade dos Santos FA, Gomes J, Alves PC, Esteves PJ, et al. +Coelho: Avaliação Ecossanitária das Populações Naturais de Coelho Bravo Visando o Controlo da Doença Hemorrágica Viral. Lisboa, Portugal: Grupo de Trabalho +Coelho. Fundo Florestal Permmanente; 2018

[116] Duarte MD, Carvalho CL, Abade dos Santos FA, Gomes J, Alves PC, Esteves PJ, et al. +Coelho 2: Desenvolvimento e implementação de medidas práticas impulsionadoras da recuperação dos leporídeos silvestres em Portugal. Lisbon: +Coelho 2 GT; 2021

[117] Dalton KP, Nicieza I, Balseiro A, Muguerza MA, Rosell JM, Casais R, et al. Variant rabbit hemorrhagic disease virus in young rabbits, Spain. Emerging Infectious Diseases. 2012;**18**(12):2009-2012

[118] Abrantes J, Lopes AM, Dalton KP, Melo P, Correia JJ, Ramada M, et al. New variant of rabbit hemorrhagic disease virus, Portugal, 2012-2013. Emerging Infectious Diseases. 2013;**19**(11):1900-1902

[119] Westcott DG, Frossard J-P, Everest D, Dastjerdi A, Duff JP, Choudhury B. Incursion of RHDV2-like variant in Great Britain. The Veterinary Record. 2014;**174**(13):333.1-333.33333. Available from: http://veterinaryrecord.bmj.com/lookup/doi/10.1136/vr.g2345

[120] Martin-Alonso A, Martin-Carrillo N, Garcia-Livia K, Valladares B, Foronda P. Emerging rabbit haemorrhagic disease virus 2 (RHDV2) at the gates of the African continent. Infection, Genetics and Evolution. 2016;**44**:46-50. Available from: http://dx.doi.org/10.1016/j.meegid.2016.06.034

[121] Hall RN, Mahar JE, Haboury S, Stevens V, Holmes EC, Strive T. Emerging rabbit hemorrhagic disease virus 2 (RHDVb), Australia. Emerging Infectious Diseases. 2015;**21**(12):2276-2278

[122] Carvalho CL, Silva S, Gouveia P, Costa M, Duarte EL, Henriques AM, et al. Emergence of rabbit haemorrhagic disease virus 2 in the archipelago of Madeira, Portugal (2016-2017). Virus Genes. 2017;**53**(6):922-926

[123] Asin J, Rejmanek D, Clifford DL, Mikolon AB, Henderson EE, Nyaoke AC, et al. Early circulation of rabbit haemorrhagic disease virus type 2 in domestic and wild lagomorphs in southern California, USA (2020-2021). Transboundary and Emerging Diseases. 2021;**69**:e394-e405

[124] Hu B, Wei H, Fan Z, Song Y, Chen M, Qiu R, et al. Emergence of rabbit haemorrhagic disease virus 2 in China in 2020. Veterinary Medicine and Science. 2021;**7**(1):236-239. Available from: https://onlinelibrary.wiley.com/doi/abs/10.1002/vms3.332

[125] Bao S, An K, Liu C, Xing X, Fu X, Xue H, et al. Rabbit hemorrhagic disease virus isolated from diseased alpine musk deer (*Moschus sifanicus*). Viruses. 2020;**12**(8):897

[126] Abade dos Santos FA, Pinto A, Burgoyne T, Dalton KP, Carvalho CL, Ramilo DW, et al. Spillover events of rabbit hemorrhagic disease virus 2 (recombinant GI.4P-GI.2) from Lagomorpha to Eurasian badger. Transboundary and Emerging Diseases. 2021;**69**(3):1030-1045

[127] Marcato PS, Benazzi C, Vecchi G, Galeotti M, Della Salda L, Sarli G, et al. Clinical and pathological features of viral haemorrhagic disease of rabbits and the European brown hare syndrome.

Revue Scientifique et Technique. 1991;**10**(2):371-392

[128] Le Gall-Recule G, Zwingelstein F, Boucher S, Le Normand B, Plassiart G, Portejoie Y, et al. Detection of a new variant of rabbit haemorrhagic disease virus in France. The Veterinary Record. 2011;**168**(5):137-138. Available from: http://veterinaryrecord.bmj.com/cgi/doi/10.1136/vr.d697

[129] Velarde R, Cavadini P, Neimanis A, Cabezón O, Chiari M, Gaffuri A, et al. Spillover events of infection of brown hares (*Lepus europaeus*) with rabbit haemorrhagic disease type 2 virus (RHDV2) caused sporadic cases of an European brown hare syndrome-like disease in Italy and Spain. Transboundary and Emerging Diseases. 2017;**64**(6):1750-1761

[130] Camarda A, Pugliese N, Cavadini P, Circella E, Capucci L, Caroli A, et al. Detection of the new emerging rabbit haemorrhagic disease type 2 virus (RHDV2) in Sicily from rabbit (*Oryctolagus cuniculus*) and Italian hare (*Lepus corsicanus*). Research in Veterinary Science. 2014;**97**(3):642-645. Available from: http://dx.doi.org/10.1016/j.rvsc.2014.10.008

[131] Neimanis A, Larsson Pettersson U, Huang N, Gavier-Widén D, Strive T. Elucidation of the pathology and tissue distribution of *Lagovirus europaeus* GI.2/RHDV2 (rabbit haemorrhagic disease virus 2) in young and adult rabbits (*Oryctolagus cuniculus*). Veterinary Research. 2018;**49**(1):1-15. Available from: https://doi.org/10.1186/s13567-018-0540-z

[132] Neimanis AS, Ahola H, Pettersson UL, Lopes AM, Abrantes J, Zohari S, et al. Overcoming species barriers: An outbreak of *Lagovirus europaeus* GI. 2/RHDV2 in an isolated population of mountain hares (*Lepus timidus*). BMC Veterinary Research. 2018;**14**(1):367

[133] OIE. Myxomatosis [Internet]. 2020. Available from: https://www.oie.int/en/animal-health-in-the-world/animal-diseases/Myxomatosis/ [Cited: 26 May 2020]

[134] Wirblich C, Meyers G, Ohlinger VF, Capucci L, Eskens U, Haas B, et al. European brown hare syndrome virus: Relationship to rabbit hemorrhagic disease virus and other caliciviruses. Journal of Virology. 1994;**68**(8):5164-5173. Available from: http://www.pubmedcentral.nih.gov/articlerender.fcgi?artid=236460&tool=pmcentrez&rendertype=abstract

[135] Gavier-Widén D, Mörner T. Descriptive epizootiological study of European brown hare syndrome in Sweden. Journal of Wildlife Diseases. 1993;**29**(1):15-20

[136] Billinis C, Psychas V, Tontis DK, Spyrou V, Birtsas PK, Sofia M, et al. European brown hare syndrome in wild European brown hares from Greece. Journal of Wildlife Diseases. 2005;**41**(4):783-786. Available from: https://doi.org/10.7589/0090-3558-41.4.783

[137] Frölich K, Fickel J, Ludwig A, Lieckfeldt D, Streich WJ, Jurčík R, et al. New variants of European brown hare syndrome virus strains in free-ranging European brown hares (*Lepus europaeus*) from Slovakia. Journal of Wildlife Diseases. 2007;**43**(1):89-96. Available from: https://doi.org/10.7589/0090-3558-43.1.89

[138] Frölich K, Meyer HHD, Pielowski Z, Ronsholt L, Seck-Lanzendorf SV, Stolte M. European brown hare syndrome in free-ranging hares in Poland. Journal of Wildlife Diseases. 1996;**32**(2):280-285. Available from: https://doi.org/10.7589/0090-3558-32.2.280

[139] Le Gall G, Huguet S, Vende P, Vautherot J-F, Rasschaert D. European

brown hare syndrome virus: Molecular cloning and sequencing of the genome. The Journal of General Virology. 1996;**77**(8):1693-1697. Available from: https://www.microbiologyresearch.org/content/journal/jgv/10.1099/0022-1317-77-8-1693

[140] Cancellotti F, Renzi M. Epidemiology and current situation of viral haemorrhagic disease of rabbits and the European brown hare syndrome in Italy. Revue Scientifique et Technique. 1991;**10**:409-422

[141] Frölich K, Haerer G, Bacciarini L, Janovsky M, Rudolph M, Giacometti M. European brown hare syndrome in free-ranging European brown and mountain hares from Switzerland. Journal of Wildlife Diseases. 2001;**37**(4):803-807

[142] Frölich K, Wisser J, Schmüser H, Fehlberg U, Neubauer H, Grunow R, et al. Epizootiologic and ecologic investigations of European brown hares (*Lepus europaeus*) in selected populations from Schleswig-Holstein, Germany. Journal of Wildlife Diseases. 2003;**39**(4):751-761

[143] Le Gall-Reculé G, Zwingelstein F, Laurent S, Portejoie Y, Rasschaert D. Molecular epidemiology of European brown hare syndrome virus in France between 1989 and 2003. Archives of Virology. 2006;**151**(9):1713-1721

[144] Gavier-Widén D, Mörner T. Epidemiology and diagnosis of the European brown hare syndrome in Scandinavian countries: A review. Revue Scientifique et Technique. 1991;**10**(2):453-458

[145] OIE. European Brown Hare Syndrome Virus (Infection with). Technical Disease Cards. Paris, France: WOAH; 2020. Available from: http://www.oie.int/wahis_2/public/wahidwild.php/Index

[146] Pellett PE, Roizman B. Herpesviridae. In: Knipe DM, Howley PM, editors. Fields Virology. 6th ed. Philadelphia, PA, USA: Wolters Kluwer; 2013. pp. 1802-1822

[147] Davison AJ, Richard E, Bernhard E, Gary HS, Duncan MJ, Anthony MC, et al. The order of Herpesvirales. Archives of Virology. 2009;**154**(1):171-177

[148] Gatherer D, Depledge DP, Hartley CA, Szpara ML, Vaz PK, Benkő M, et al. ICTV virus taxonomy profile: Herpesviridae 2021. The Journal of General Virology. 2021;**102**(10):1673. Available from: https://www.microbiologyresearch.org/content/journal/jgv/10.1099/jgv.0.001673

[149] David M. Knipe PM. Fields Virology. In: Knipe DM, Howley PM, editors. Fields Virology. 6th ed. Philadelphia, PA, USA: Lippincott Williams & Wilkins; 2013. p. 2456

[150] Jin L, Löhr CV, Vanarsdall AL, Baker RJ, Moerdyk-Schauwecker M, Levine C, et al. Characterization of a novel alphaherpesvirus associated with fatal infections of domestic rabbits. Virology. 2008;**378**(1):13-20

[151] Sunohara-Neilson JR, Brash M, Carman S, Nagy É, Turner PV. Experimental infection of New Zealand white rabbits (*Oryctolagus cuniculi*) with leporid herpesvirus 4. Comparative Medicine. 2013;**63**(5):422-431

[152] Barthold SW, Griffey SM, Percy DH. Rabbit. In: Pathology of Laboratory Rodents and Rabbits. 4th ed. Nova Jersey, EUA: John Wiley & Sons, Ltd.; 2016. p. 258

[153] Abade dos Santos FA, Monteiro M, Pinto A, Carvalho CL, Peleteiro MC, Carvalho P, et al. First description of a herpesvirus infection in genus *Lepus*. PLoS One. 2020;**15**(4):e0231795.

Available from: https://pubmed.ncbi.nlm.nih.gov/32302375

[154] Roizmanm B, Furlong D. The replication of herpesviruses. In: Fraenkel-Conrat H, editor. Comprehensive Virology. New York: Plenum Press; 1974. pp. 229-403

[155] Falke D, Siegert R, Vogell W. Electron microscopic findings on the problem of double membrane formation in herpes simplex virus. Archiv für die Gesamte Virusforschung. 1959;**9**:484-496

[156] Armstrong JA, Pereira HG, Andrewes CH. Observations on the virus of infectious bovine rhinotracheitis, and its affinity with the Herpesvirus group. Virology. 1961;**14**:276-285

[157] Furlong D, Swift H, Roizman B. Arrangement of herpesvirus deoxyribonucleic acid in the core. Journal of Virology. 1972;**10**(5):1071-1074

[158] Booy FP, Trus BL, Davison AJ, Steven AC. The capsid architecture of channel catfish virus, an evolutionarily distant herpesvirus, is largely conserved in the absence of discernible sequence homology with herpes simplex virus. Virology. 1996;**215**(2):134-141

[159] Davison AJ, Trus BL, Cheng N, Steven AC, Watson MS, Cunningham C, et al. A novel class of herpesvirus with bivalve hosts. The Journal of General Virology. 2005;**86**(Pt 1):41-53

[160] Liu F, Zhou ZH. Chapter 3—Comparative virion structures of human herpesviruses. In: Arvin A, Campadelli-Fiume G, Mocarski E, Moore PS, Roizman B, Whitley R, et al., editors. Human Herpesviruses: Biology, Therapy, and Immunoprophylaxis. Cambridge: Cambridge University Press; 2007. pp. 27-43

[161] Gibson W. Structure and assembly of the virion. Intervirology. 1996;**39**(5-6):389-400

[162] Mettenleiter TC. Intriguing interplay between viral proteins during herpesvirus assembly or: The herpesvirus assembly puzzle. Veterinary Microbiology. 2006;**113**(3-4):163-169

[163] Marlier D. Vaccination strategies against myxomavirus infections: Are we really doing the best? Tijdschrift voor Diergeneeskunde. 2010;**135**(5):194-198

[164] Joubert L, Leftheriosis E, Mouchet J. La Myxomatose (in French) [Internet]. Lepine P, Goret P, editors. L' Expansion Scientifique Française. Vol. 84. No. 643. 1972. pp. 487-492. Available from: http://ir.obihiro.ac.jp/dspace/handle/10322/3933

[165] Brun A, Saurat P, Gilbert Y, Godart A, Bouquet JF. Données actuelles sur l'épidémiologie, la pathogénie et la symptomatologie de la myxomatose. Revue De Medecine Veterinaire. 1981;**132**:585-590

[166] Ferreira C, Ramírez E, Castro F, Ferreras P, Alves PC, Redpath S, et al. Field experimental vaccination campaigns against myxomatosis and their effectiveness in the wild. Vaccine. 2009;**27**(50):6998-7002

[167] Guitton J-S, Devillard S, Guénézan M, Fouchet D, Pontier D, Marchandeau S. Vaccination of free-living juvenile wild rabbits (*Oryctolagus cuniculus*) against myxomatosis improved their survival. Preventive Veterinary Medicine. 2008;**84**(1-2):1-10

[168] Arthur CP, Louzis C. A review of myxomatosis among rabbits in France. Revue Scientifique et Technique. 1988;7(4):959-976

[169] Fenner F, Woodroof GM. Protection of laboratory rabbits against myxomatosis by vaccination with fibroma virus. The Australian Journal of Experimental Biology and Medical Science. 1954;**32**(5):653-668

[170] Saito JK, McKercher DG, Castrucci G. Attenuation of the myxoma virus and use of the living attenuated virus as an immunizing agent for myxomatosis. The Journal of Infectious Diseases. 1964;**114**(5):417-428. Available from: https://doi.org/10.1093/infdis/114.5.417

[171] Rosell JM, Fuente L, Parra F, Dalton K, Sáiz J, de Rozas A, et al. Myxomatosis and rabbit haemorrhagic disease: A 30-year study of the occurrence on commercial farms in Spain. Animals. 2019;**9**:780

[172] Dalton KP, Nicieza I, De LD, Gullón J, Inza M, Petralanda M, et al. Vaccine breaks: Outbreaks of myxomatosis on Spanish commercial rabbit farms. Veterinary Microbiology. 2015;**178**(3-4): 208-216. Available from: http://dx.doi.org/10.1016/j.vetmic.2015.05.008

[173] Flowerdew JR, Trout RC, Ross J. Myxomatosis: Population dynamics of rabbits (*Oryctolagus cuniculus* Linnaeus, 1758) and ecological effects in the United Kingdom. Revue Scientifique et Technique. 1992;**11**(4):1109-1113

[174] Trout RC, Ross J, Tittensor AM, Fox AP. The effect on a British wild rabbit population (*Oryctolagus cuniculus*) of manipulating myxomatosis. Journal of Applied Ecology. 1992;**29**(3):679-686. Available from: http://www.jstor.org/stable/2404476

[175] García-Bocanegra I, Camacho-Sillero L, Risalde MA, Dalton K, Caballero-Gómez J, Aguero M, et al. First outbreak of myxomatosis in Iberian hares (*Lepus granatensis*). Transboundary and Emerging Diseases. 2019;**66**(6):2204-2208

[176] Hernández Ó, Sánchez-García C, Tizado EJ. Impact of myxomatosis on densities of Iberian hares (*Lepus granatensis*) in North-Western Spain: Implications for management and sustainable hunting. The European Zoological Journal. 2022;**89**(1):204-209. Available from: https://doi.org/10.1080/24750263.2022.2037759

[177] Williams RT, Dunsmore JD, Parer I. Evidence for the existence of latent myxoma virus in rabbits (*Oryctolagus cuniculus* (L.)). Nature. 1972;**238**(5359):99-101. Available from: https://doi.org/10.1038/238099a0

[178] Carvalho CL, Abade dos Santos FA, Fagulha T, Carvalho P, Mendonça P, Monteiro M, et al. Myxoma virus and rabbit haemorrhagic disease virus 2 coinfection in a European wild rabbit (*Oryctolagus cuniculus* algirus), Portugal. Veterinary Record Case Reports. 2020;**8**(1):18-21

[179] Soriguer R, Carro F. *Lepus granatensis*. The IUCN Red List of Threatened Species. 2019:e. T41306A2953195. DOI: 10.2305/IUCN.UK.2019-1.RLTS.T41306A2953195.en. [Accessed: 11 March 2023]

[180] WWF. Living Planet Report 2020—Bending the curve of biodiversity loss. In: Almond REA, Grooten M, Petersen T, editors. Gland, Switzerland: WWF; 2020. ISBN 978-2-940529-99-5

Section 4

Viral Outbreaks Linked to Fish

Chapter 7

Status of Emerging and Reemerging Fish Viral Infections in India

Kollanoor Riji John, Panchavarnam Sivasankar and Mulloorpeedikayil Rosalind George

Abstract

Aquaculture, being the fastest growing food production sector, has now become vital to the socioeconomic development of many countries. In India, aquaculture plays a significant role in food production, ensuring nutritional security, boosting agricultural exports, and generating job opportunities. The production of farmed fish has greatly expanded qualitatively and quantitatively in both freshwater and marine water regimes to fulfill the ever-growing demand. However, the occurrence of diseases is the main obstacle to sustainable aquaculture production, which has an impact on the socioeconomic status of fish farmers of the country. Viral diseases inflict irreparable damage to the aquaculture enterprise causing large-scale economic losses and ecological problems. Recently, there has been a spike in the incidence of new emerging viral diseases in diverse species of aquaculture species. Prophylactics by far being the only feasible method of viral disease control, the development of viral vaccines is highly imperative. A precise understanding of the disease pathology, etiological agent, and species susceptible to the specific diseases are highly essential in this perspective. The chapter highlights the emerging and reemerging viral diseases in the Indian aquaculture sector.

Keywords: aquaculture, disease emergence, virus occurrence, fish

1. Introduction

Aquaculture is one of the fastest food-producing sectors in the world that contributes significantly to the world economy. World aquaculture production has increased from 35.6 million tonnes in 2000 to 87.5 million tonnes in 2020 (**Figure 1**). At present, India is the third largest fish-producing country in the world and accounts for 7.96% of the global production. Fish production increased from 5.66 MMT in FY2000–2001 to 8.67 MMT in FY2011–2012. During FY2020–2021, the total production has been estimated at 14.73 MMT with the contribution of 11.25 MMT from inland sector and 3.48 MMT from marine sector. Indian aquaculture production during 2000–2020 ranged from about 2 million tonnes to 8.7 million tonnes in 2020 (**Figure 2**). In India, fish culture encompasses a diverse range of fishes, including Indian major carps,

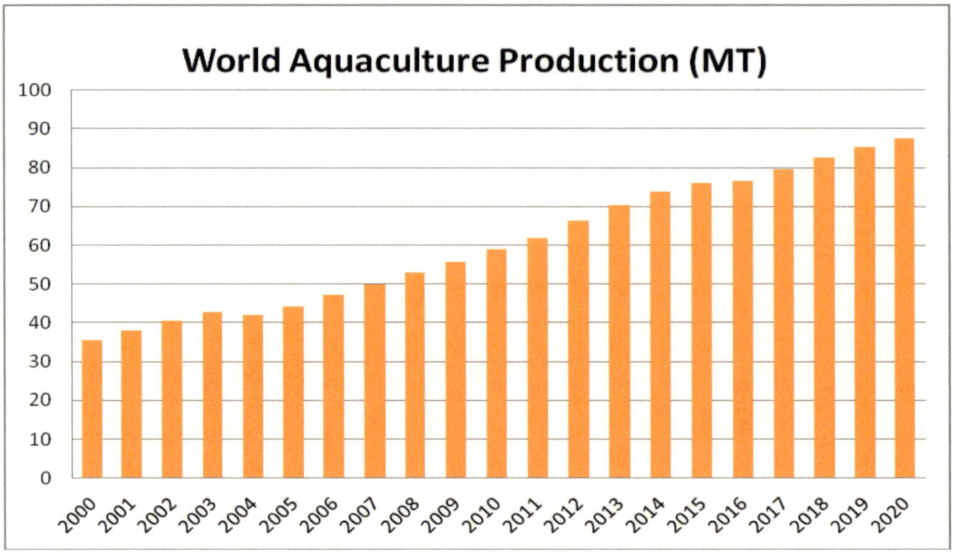

Figure 1.
World aquatic animal production increased from 35.5 million tonnes in 2000 to 87.5 million tonnes in 2020 (Source: FAO 2000–2022).

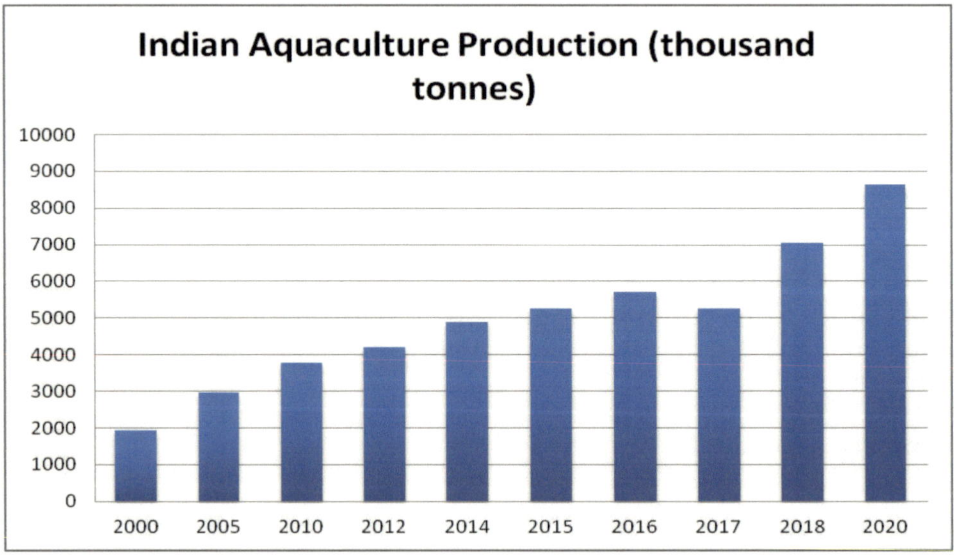

Figure 2.
Indian aquaculture production reached from 1943 thousand tonnes in 2000 to 8641.3 thousand tonnes in 2020 (Source: FAO 2000–2022).

minor carps, catfishes, barbs, tilapia, climbing perch, and murrels. Additionally, due to the esthetic value and economic benefit of ornamental fish farming, it has become more and more popular throughout the world. In India, ornamental fish farming is mainly practiced in West Bengal, Tamil Nadu, Kerala, Karnataka, and states of the North East [1], and the country possesses great potential in contributing to the global ornamental sectors [2].

Intensification of aquaculture has increased productivity significantly while concurrently accompanied with several infectious diseases. Successful aquaculture production relies on various factors like stocking density, pond management, and development of the host immune system.

Health management in aquatic animals requires more attention and care for monitoring and control than terrestrial counterparts. Intensive aquaculture, in particular, has brought in more disease problems due to infectious agents, some of which are difficult to control and lead to high economic losses. By far viral diseases are found to be more difficult to control than bacterial and fungal diseases.

Until the 1980s, marine viruses were considered ecologically insignificant, because their concentrations were underestimated, but subsequent studies have confirmed that the ocean contains an abundance of organisms, including millions of virus particles per milliliter of seawater [3]. Most of the fish diseases, however, can be controlled by proper scientific management through appropriate biosecurity, nutritional adequacy, prophylactics, water and sediment quality control, adequate aeration, checking, and controlling input quality including fish seed, feed and chemicals, and constant monitoring through sampling.

New or previously unknown diseases; known diseases appearing for the first time in a new species; known diseases appearing for the first time in a new location; and known diseases with a new sign or higher virulence may be considered as emerging diseases [4]. This article provides a thorough insight into some of the important viral pathogens that are emerging and reemerging fish viruses in Indian aquaculture. Additionally, it provides current diagnostic techniques and disease control methods, as well as future directions for preventing potential diseases in wild and farmed fish.

2. Common disease problems in Indian aquaculture

Infectious diseases are the major constraints to aquaculture and the limiting factor for economic and socioeconomic development of fish farmers in India and many other countries in the world [5–7]. Some diseases have seriously affected the future development of the aquaculture sector as well as the livelihood of fish farmers. Intensification of cultural practices without the fundamental understanding of the complex balance between host, pathogen, and environment has led to many diseases that threaten present-day aquaculture [8, 9]. In India, the expansion of aquaculture into intensive and semi-intensive methods has been accompanied by an increase in production of fish and shellfish due to high stocking densities. However, stressful environmental circumstances encourage the emergence and spread of infectious diseases through variations in virulence and epidemiological factors [10]. Infectious diseases, especially viral diseases are very difficult to be controlled once established within the culture system [11] due to the peculiar environment where pathogens are constantly lurking for an opportunity when the health status of the host is compromised [12]. Many diseases in aquaculture are directly correlated with environmental deterioration including non-optimal water quality, higher microbial load, and poor nutritional status which leads to stress to the cultured animals. In addition, opportunistic pathogens present in the aquatic environment become harmful due to high stocking density [13]. Many new diseases have emerged in fish and shrimp culture as a result of expansion of the aquaculture sector, increased global movement of aquatic animals and their products, and various anthropogenic interventions in the ecosystem that lead to stress to aquatic animals.

3. Emerging viral diseases of finfish

In India, indigenous major caps (IMC) namely, catla, rohu, mrigal; exotic carps like common carp, grass carp, silver carp along with catfishes (*Clarius batrachus, Heteropneuestes fossilis, Pangassius* spp.) and freshwater prawn *Macrobrachium rosenbergii* are widely cultured. The culture of pacu, *Piaractus brachypomus*, and the exotic catfish *Pangasiandon hypophthalamus* has also grown during the past few years. Additionally, Tilapia and Pangasius offer great potential for cage culture in freshwater lakes and reservoirs [13]. Several diseases caused by viruses have been identified in fish all over the world. However, there have only been a few instances of viral diseases affecting finfish in India. Viral diseases due to Koi ranavirus (KIRV), Similar damselfish virus (SRDV), Red sea bream iridovirus (RSIV), Infectious spleen and kidney necrosis virus (ISKNV), Carp edema virus (CEV), Viral Nervous Necrosis (LCNNV-In), Tilapia Lake Virus (TiLV), and Snakehead rhabdovirus (SHRV-In) have been reported in India.

3.1 Iridoviruses

3.1.1 Koi ranavirus (KIRV)

In India, a ranavirus infecting koi (KIRV) was reported for the first time in 2015, which was isolated and characterized from moribund koi (*Cyprinus carpio*) that suffered continuous mortality exhibiting swimming abnormalities, intermittent surfacing, and skin darkening (**Figure 3**) [14]. Icosahedral virus particles of 100–120 nm were observed in the infected cell cultures, budding from the cell membrane (**Figure 4**). Sequence analysis of the major capsid protein gene showed an identity of 99.9% to that of the largemouth bass virus isolated from North America.

Iridoviruses are double-stranded DNA viruses having icosahedral capsid with a size range of about 120–200 nm and a genome size ranging from 102 to 210 kbp [15]. The family Iridoviridae is subdivided into five genera, the Iridovirus and Chloriridovirus genera that infect insects, the Lymphocystivirus and Megalocytivirus genera, which

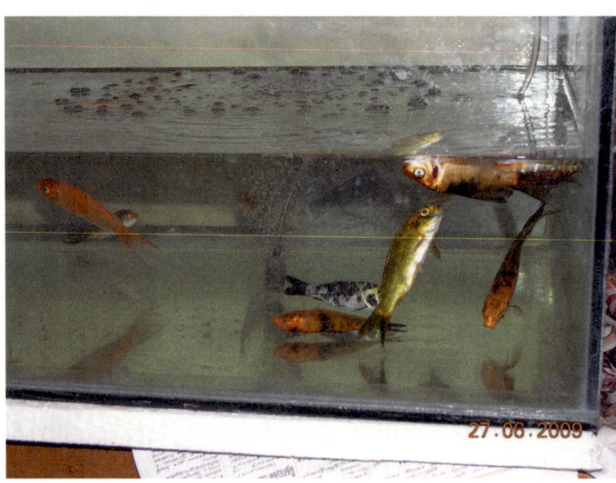

Figure 3.
Koi infected with koi ranavirus (KIRV) showing clinical signs such as skin darkening, loss of scales, vertical hanging, uncoordinated swimming, turning upside down, lateral rotation, intermittent surfacing, and settling at the bottom.

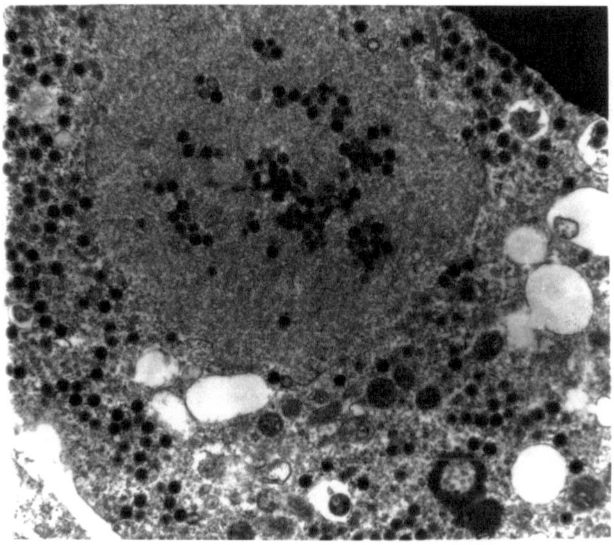

Figure 4.
Transmission electron micrographs of koi ranavirus (KIRV) in snakehead kidney (SNKD2a) cells showing icosahedral particle of 100–120 nm size.

infect fish species and Ranavirus, which are genetically diverse and infect amphibians, fish, and reptiles [16]. Ranaviruses can cause acute, systemic disease in fish with increasing severity resulting from necrosis of kidney and spleen and hemorrhages on the skin and internal organs [16, 17]. Viruses of the genera Ranavirus are of growing concern to aquaculture owing to their ability to cause large-scale mortality in a wide variety of host species [17–20]. The common clinical signs of KIRV-infected fishes were uncoordinated swimming, rolling over, and vertical hanging before death [14].

Some iridovirus strains such as epizootic hematopoietic necrosis virus (EHNV) occur in apparently healthy fish without any clinical, indicating the carrier state. Experimental infection with EHNV also results in seroconversion in Australian frogs *Bufo marinus* without any clinical disease signs [21]. Type species FV3 of the genus Ranavirus differs from several other ranaviruses reported. Ranaviruses infect multiple cold-blooded vertebrates and have been found to undergo several host shifts suggesting the possibility of these viruses crossing the poikilothermic species barriers leading eventually to potentially devastating diseases in new hosts [22]. Molecular analysis based on the nucleotide sequences of the major capsid protein (MCP), DNA polymerase, and neurofilament triplet H1-like (NF-H1) protein gene distinguished two tropical ranavirus isolates, guppy virus 6 (GV6) and doctor fish virus (DFV) from European and Australian ranavirus isolates [23]. However, these two viruses were found to be very similar but not identical with the North American Santee-Cooper ranavirus isolated from largemouth bass [24] and KIRV [14], which had 99.21% sequence homogeneity between them for 1123 bp MCP fragment. Due to the phylogenetic variations, it is suggested that the Santee-Cooper ranavirus and related viruses such as the doctor fish virus and guppy virus may not belong to the genus [25, 26]. The presence of ranavirus was again found in carps (*Puntius sarana* and *Osteobrama belangeri*) that had extensive mortality in North East India in 2016 [27]. The sequence analysis of the 321 bp fragment has shown 98.9% homology with the major capsid protein gene of KIRV that was detected from south India [14].

3.1.2 Similar damselfish virus (SRDV)

Similar damselfish virus was isolated and characterized from marine ornamental "Similar Damselfish" (*Pomacentrus similis* Allen, 1991) in India in 2017 [28]. The virus was identified as a member of the genus *Ranavirus* of the family *Iridoviridae*. SRDV grows well in marine and freshwater fish cell lines from seabass and snakehead. It is a large and icosahedral virus of 120–130 nm having double-stranded DNA genome. Experimental infection of similar damselfish fingerlings with the SRDV showed cumulative mortalities up to 93.33%. SRDV infected fish were found to exhibit clinical signs such as skin discoloration and ulcer, lethargy, anorexia, sudden jerky movement, circling around the central axis, and settling at the bottom of the tank before mortality [28]. Phylogenetically, the virus had 99.82% identity with largemouth bass virus and 99.29% identity with KIRV across 1130 MCP fragment. Partial cross-neutralization was observed between recently isolated ranaviruses, SRDV, and KIRV against SRDV antisera indicating similarity among the immunogenic epitopes of the capsid proteins.

3.1.3 Red sea bream iridovirus (RSIV)

The red sea bream iridovirus (RSIV) is a member of the Megalocytivirus genus which causes severe mortality in farm-reared red sea bream (*Pagrus major*). RSIV infection also occurs in more than 30 other species of farmed marine fish [29, 30]. First recorded in Japan in 1990, the disease is widely distributed in several Asian countries including Taiwan, China, Hong Kong, Korea, Japan, Malaysia, Singapore, and Thailand [31]. In India, the emergence of RSIV infection was first reported in cultured Asian seabass in 2019 [32]. Affected fish were lethargic, exhibited severe anemia, petechiae of the gills, and enlargement of the spleen [33]. Histopathological changes such as increased RBC proliferation, lymphocytic infiltration, fused secondary lamellae, necrosed cellular material, and reduced secondary lamellae height was observed in RSIV-infected gill tissue. Additionally, leucocytic depopulation in the white pulp, melanomacrophage centers, increased vacuoles, and irregular intracytoplasmic viral inclusion bodies could be found in RSIV infected spleen. This virus caused 100% mortality in experimentally challenged seabass within 6 days of post-infection [32]. For RSIVD control, an effective formalin-killed vaccine was developed and is now commercially available for red sea bream (*P. major*), striped jack (*Pseudocaranx dentex*), Malabar grouper (*Epinephelus malabaricus*), orange-spotted grouper (*Epinephelus coioides*), and other fish species belonging to the genus Seriola in Japan. Complete genome analysis of the Indian strain of RSIV showed that the virus has a 111,557 bp genome and belongs to RSIV-Genotype II [34].

3.1.4 Infectious spleen and kidney necrosis virus (ISKNV)

Infectious spleen and kidney necrosis virus (ISKNV) is a type of species of the genus *Megalocytivirus* under the family *Iridoviridae* [35]. ISKNV was first detected in 1994 in the Chinese mandarin fish *Siniperca chuatsi*, that resulted in severe economic losses [36, 37]. Later, it was found spread other countries like Korea, Malaysia, Indonesia, Singapore, Australia, and Germany. The virus was reported in India in 2020 causing infection in a wide range of ornamental fish species [38]. The virus has a vast host range and can infect nearly 50 different freshwater, brackishwater, and marine species [39]. Among the popular freshwater ornamental fish species, cichlids such as the angelfish *Pterophyllum scalare*, livebearers, and some gourami species are susceptible to ISKNV [40].

ISKNV-infected fish showed anorexia, petechial hemorrhages, abnormal swimming, and pale coloration [37]. Gross changes included swelling of the kidneys and spleen. Histopathologically, hypertrophic cells with large basophilic cytoplasmic inclusions were found in the spleen, kidney, gill tissue, cranial connective tissue, and the endocardium [37]. Experimental infection of pearl gourami *Trichogaster leeri* and silver gourami *T. microlepis* with a tissue homogenate of pearl gourami infected by ISKNV induced 70% and 20% cumulative mortalities in the pearl and silver gourami, respectively [41]. ISKNV caused significant mortalities of ornamental fish species in India during the year 2018–2019 with various clinical signs such as erratic swimming, sluggish movement, fin rot, hemorrhage, mucus secretion, and body discoloration [32].

3.1.5 Lymphocystis disease virus (LCDV)

Lymphocystis virus disease affects a large number of freshwater, brackish water, and marine fish species across the world. LCD is characterized by epithelial benign tumors resulting from hypertrophied fibroblast connective cells of the body and fins. Presence of epidermal papilloma like benign tumor used to appear on farm-reared adult grass carp, *Ctenopharyngodon idella* in the northern part of India during the winter months (November–January) of 2017–2019. Investigation was the first report of the occurrence of lymphocystis disease in grass carp in India [42]. The viral agent was identified as LCDV LRI-18 following molecular and histological identification techniques. Phylogenetic examination of the partial nucleotide sequence of LCDV DNA polymerase gene revealed close relatedness of LCDV LRI-18 (GenBank No. MK347473) and the LCDV strain from Israel, sharing 99.0% and 96.5% homology among the respective nucleotide and amino acid sequences.

Single or multiple intracytoplasmic inclusion bodies have been noticed on lymphocystis and erythrocyte cells of grass carp infected with LCDV LRI-18. The virions were icosahedral in shape with an electron-dense core and had a size of 280 nm diameter [42]. Histopathologically, LCDV-infected grass carp had extensive hypertrophy and lamellar fusion, hemorrhage in the eye, liver necrosis, myocardial inflammation, fused intestinal villi, and glomerular degeneration. Experimental dip infection in 0.45 m filtered LCDV crude suspension did not reproduce the disease in grass carp fingerlings., and also no death was noted.

3.2 Carp edema virus (CEV)

Carp edema virus disease (CEVD) is an emerging disease of concern to koi enthusiasts and carp aquaculture around the world. Carp edema virus is a large, double-stranded DNA virus belonging to the poxvirus family of viruses (*Poxviridae*). Carp edema virus disease/koi sleepy disease differs widely from another similar disease referred to as “carp pox,” which is caused by a herpesvirus (Cyprinid herpesvirus 1) that is responsible for wart-like growths on the skin in common carp varieties [43]. The CEV was first detected in Japanese koi in the 1970s and derived its name from causing edematous skin lesions in the affected fish [44]. The infection of CEV has been reported in three continents, Asia, North America, and Europe, particularly from Germany, India, China, Korea, and Iraq from common carp and koi carp [45]. The infection with CEV was reported in India for the first time in koi that was showing clinical signs similar to sleepy disease [45]. Of late, large-scale mortality caused by CEV in koi carps (*C. carpio koi*) has been found in the ornamental fish farm of Odisha, India [46].

Common carp (*C. carpio*), especially koi, can contract the carp edema virus, which can lead to disease and high mortality rates. The disease was formerly known as "viral edema of carp" because sick fish may have erosive or hemorrhagic skin lesions along with swelling (edema) of the underlying tissues (**Figure 5**) [47]. The infected fish could also exhibit the clinical signs of ulcers on body, massive necrosis of gills, and sleeping at the bottom of tanks before death (**Figure 6**) [45]. In the early stages of the disease, the gill epithelial cells at the tips of the gill filament proliferate, resulting in a thickening or "clubbing" appearance (**Figure 7**) [48]. In CEV-infected fish, the proliferation may extend to the base of the gill filament and impair gill function. Common carp and koi (*C. carpio*) are the only known susceptible species [49].

The disease is also known as "koi sleepy sickness" (KSD) due to the strange behavior of affected fish, which includes being unresponsive and lethargic and frequently

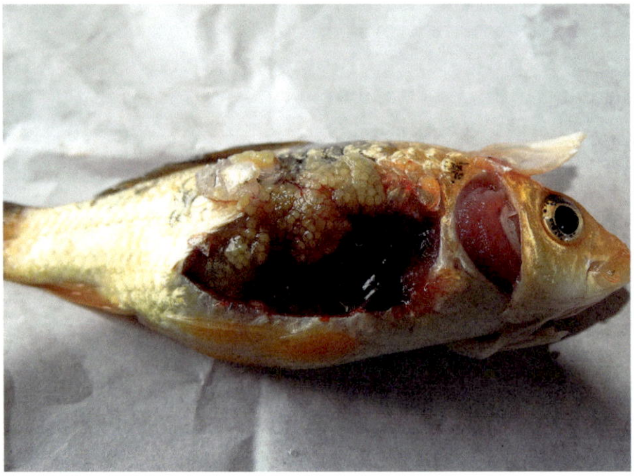

Figure 5.
Koi infected with carp edema virus having dropsy showing internal hemorrhage and serosanguinous fluid in the peritoneal cavity.

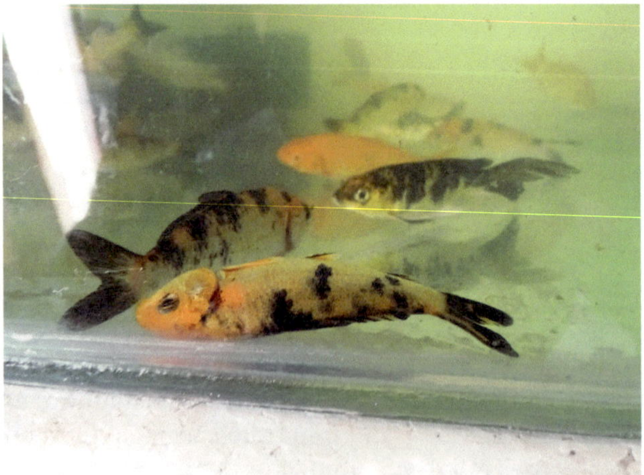

Figure 6.
CEV infected the clinical signs of ulcers on body, massive necrosis of gills, and sleeping at the bottom of tanks before death.

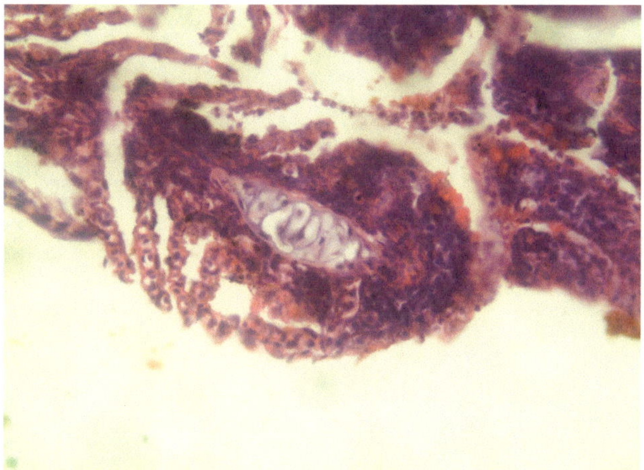

Figure 7.
CEV-infected koi gill epithelial cells proliferated at the tips of the gill filament, resulting in lamellar fusion and thickening or "clubbing" appearance.

lying motionless at the tank floor for extended periods of time if undisturbed. Once the "sleepy" carp is disturbed, they swim for a little while and soon become passive and settle on the tank's bottom [48]. The severity of the disease is greatest in juveniles, which may hang just under the surface of the water before succumbing, while adult fish may lie motionless on the bottom of the pond/tank [49].

3.3 Viral nervous necrosis (VNN)

Fish nodaviruses, members of the genus *Betanodavirus* under the family *Nodaviridae*, are the causative agents of a highly destructive disease in approximately 150 species of marine finfish species worldwide [50]. Following the first outbreak of the viral nervous necrosis disease at early larval stage in seabass hatcheries in Martinique, the French Mediterranean [51] and Queensland [52], the causative agent was first identified as a member of the family *Nodaviridae* by molecular analysis of the purified virus from infected hatchery-reared larvae of striped jack *P. dentex* [53]. Viral nervous necrosis (VNN), also known as viral encephalopathy and retinopathy (VER), is a disease caused by nodaviruses, which are icosahedral in shape having a size range of 25–34 nm (**Figure 8**). The virus has a single-stranded bipartite positive sense RNA genome. Although adults can be affected, hatchery-reared larvae and juveniles are primarily affected by VNN outbreaks, which can cause high mortalities of up to 100% [54]. The virus was first isolated in cell culture from seabass fry using striped snakehead cell line [55]. There are four genotypes recognized under the genus including red-spotted grouper nervous necrosis virus (RGNNV), barfin flounder nervous necrosis virus (BFNNV), tiger puffer nervous necrosis virus (TPNNV), and striped jack nervous necrosis virus (SJNNV) based on the comparative sequence analyses of the coat protein genes [56].

The VNN has been reported in many countries including Southeast Asia (India, Indonesia, China, Japan, Korea, Malaysia, Philippines, Thailand, and Vietnam), Oceania (Australia, Tahiti), the Mediterranean Basin (France, Greece, Italy, Malta, Portugal, Spain, and Tunisia), the UK, Norway, the Caribbean Islands, and North America (USA and Canada) [50, 57]. In India, betanodavirus infection has been observed in both cultured and wild population of brackishwater/marine

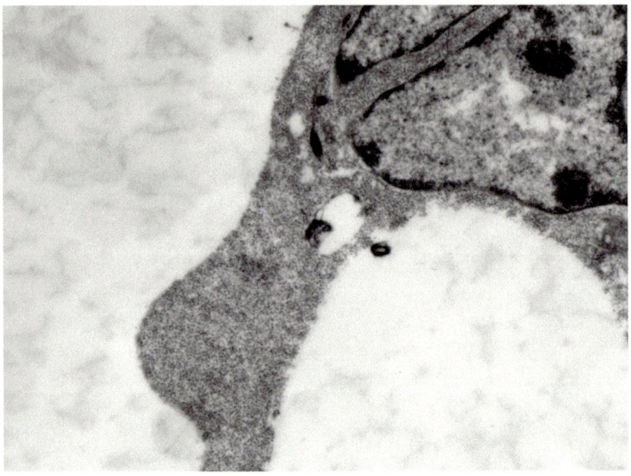

Figure 8.
Transmission electron micrographs of Lates calcarifer nervous necrosis nodavirus in SSN1 cell line.

fish species (**Figure 9**) such as *Lates calcarifer, Rachycentron canadum, Trachinotus blochii, Mugil cephalus, Liza parsia, Chanos chanos, Epinephelus tauvina, Sardinella longiceps, Amblygaster clupeoides, Thrissocles dussumieri, Leiognathus splendens, Upeneus sulphureus,* and *Mystus gulio* (reviewed by Jithendran et al. [58]. In addition, the infection has also been recorded among aquarium fishes including *Carassius auratus* (Gold fish), *Epalzeorhynchos frenatum* (Rainbow shark), *Danio rerio* (Zebra fish) and *Amphiprion sebae* (Clown fish) [58]. *Betanodavirus* genotypes show different optimal growth temperatures, 15–20°C for BFNNV, 20°C for TPNNV, 20–25°C for SJNNV, and 25–30°C for RGNNV [59]. The temperature sensitivity of betanodaviruses seems to be regulated by the region encoding the amino acid residues 1–445 of RNA1 [59].

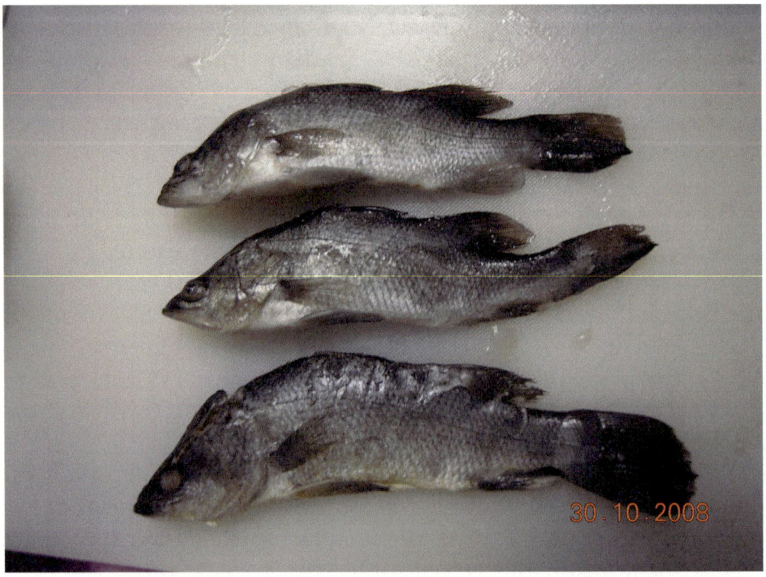

Figure 9.
Viral nervous necrosis (NNV)-infected juvenile seabass.

Clinical signs due to VNN infection depend on the fish species, biological stage, phase of the disease, and temperature. However, common signs are abnormal swimming behavior (spiral swimming, whirling, horizontal looping, or darting) and loss of appetite among affected fish [60, 61]. Other signs include swim bladder hyperinflation and coloration abnormalities (pale or dark). Histopathologically, the fish show extensive necrosis of the central nervous system (CNS), with extensive vacuolation and neural degeneration of the brain as well as vacuolation of the retina [60–62]. The main clinical signs of NNV infection in freshwater fish include anorexia, descaling, and settling the bottom with dropsy [58]. An experimental infection performed using guppy (*Poecilia reticulata*) showed clear clinical signs associated with significant mortality since 15 dpi [63]. The cumulative mortalities reached up to 100% at 30 dpi in the study. A pathogenicity study in seabass fingerlings using betanodavirus revealed nervous necrosis in retinal cells following a 21-day challenge trial (**Figure 10**) [64]. Both horizontal and vertical transmission has been demonstrated in several fish species [50].

3.4 Tilapia lake virus (TiLV)

Tilapia Lake Virus (TiLV) disease is an emerging and transboundary disease of tilapia, causing mortality up to 90% globally in farmed tilapia over the last 4–5 years [65, 66]. TiLV is an enveloped, negative-sense, single-stranded RNA virus (-ssRNA) with a 10,323 kb genome and a size range of 55–100 nm diameter [65]. It was first identified as an orthomyxo-like virus and the only member of the genus *Tilapinevirus* in the family *Amnoonviridae* [65, 67, 68]. Until 2009, there were no reports on viral diseases in Tilapia. However, large-scale mortalities were seen in both wild and farmed hybrid tilapia (*Oreochromis niloticus* × *O. aureus*) in Israel during the summer of 2009, the etiological agent of which was identified as Tilapia Lake Virus (TiLV) in 2013 [65]. Further, outbreaks of TiLV have been reported from other countries

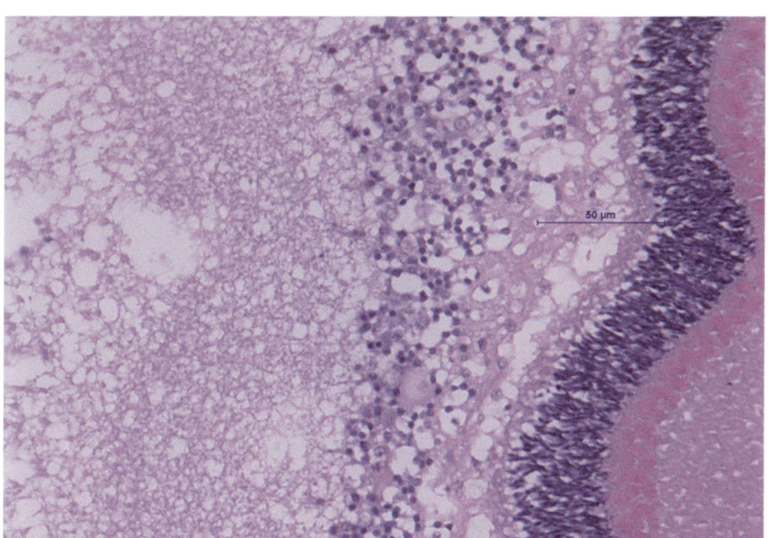

Figure 10.
H&E stained section of the retina of experimentally infected seabass juveniles showing extensive vacuolation of the cells in outer plexifrom and inner nuclear layer. Photo courtesy: Lekshmi Haridas.

namely, Ecuador, Colombia, Egypt, Thailand, Chinese Taipei, Malaysia, Bangladesh, Uganda, Tanzania, Peru, Mexico, Philippines, Indonesia, and USA. In India, TiLV was first reported following the outbreaks of a fatal disease in farmed tilapia in two states, West Bengal and Kerala [69].

There are several clinical signs associated with TiLV; however, corneal opacity may be one of the overt clinical signs of TiLV infection [65]. The infected fishes could exhibit other signs like anorexia, poor body condition, severe anemia, bilateral exophthalmia, skin abrasion and congestion, scale protrusion, and abdominal swelling (**Figure 11**) [70–72]. In addition, clinical signs like pale coloration of the body, gathering at the bottom, sluggish movement, abnormal swimming, and avoidance of schooling before death have also been observed during the outbreak [73]. The brain and liver are the most targeted organs for TiLV infection [66]. Histopathological changes in the liver are characterized by hepatic syncytia and thus the name "syncytial hepatitis" (**Figure 12**). Pathologies in the brain included blood vessel congestion and infiltration of lymphocytes, which have been associated with the clinical sign of irregular swimming [74]. Recently, co-infection of bacteria, *Lactococcus garvieae* with TiLV and associated mass mortality in Nile tilapia was reported in India [75].

3.5 Snakehead rhabdovirus

Rhabdoviruses and aquabirnaviruses are among the most potentially harmful viral pathogens of fishes. The family *Rhabdoviridae* comprises bullet-shaped enveloped viruses that are classified into 18 genera and 134 species (**Figure 13**) [76]. Rhabdoviruses have an enveloped virion with the nucleocapsid (30–70 nm in diameter) containing a single molecule of linear, negative-sense ssRNA genomes of 10–16 kb size, which encodes five virion structural proteins: the nucleoprotein (N), the phosphoprotein (P), the matrix protein (M), the glycoprotein (G), and the polymerase (L) [77]. Rhabdoviruses infecting fish are included in the genera *Novirhabdovirus,*

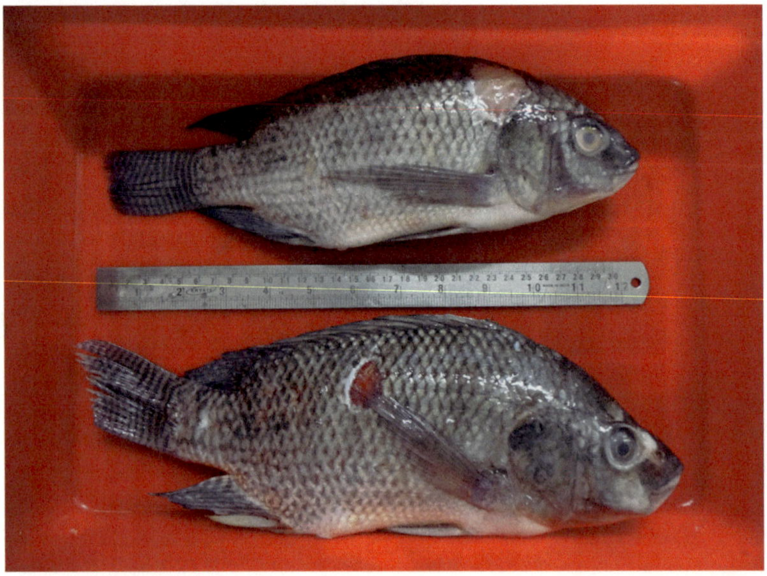

Figure 11.
TiLV-infected tilapia showing exophthalmia, hemorrhages, skin ulcers swollen abdomen, and eroded fins.

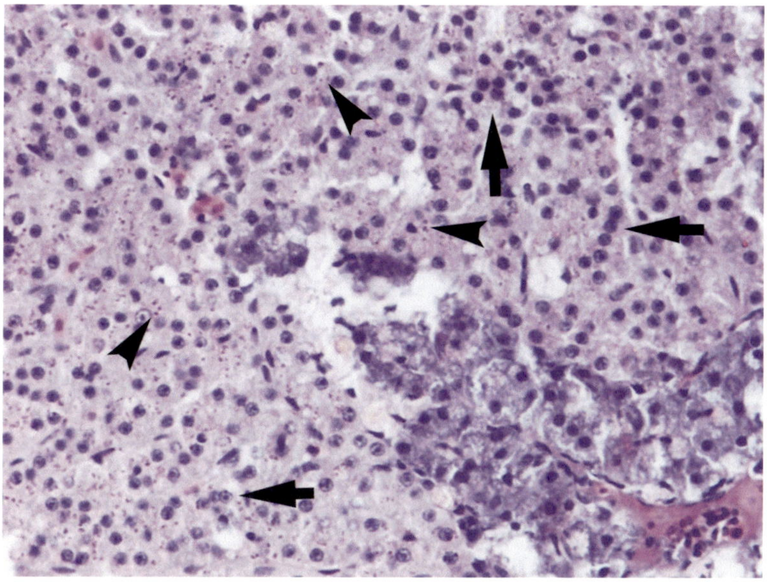

Figure 12.
Histopathological section of TiLV-infected liver stained in hematoxylin and eosin showing putative intracytoplasmic inclusion body (arrowhead) with giant cell having multiple nuclei (arrow). Photo courtesy: Lekshmi Haridas.

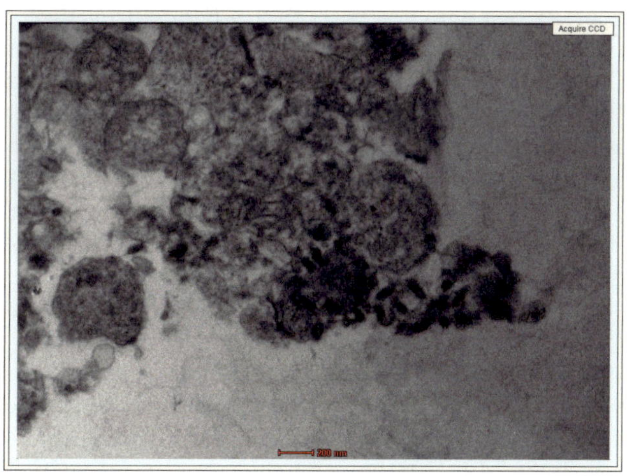

Figure 13.
Transmission electron micrographs of snakehead rhabdovirus particles (SHRV-In) in the virus-infected SSN1 cells revealing bullet-shaped virus particles (bar 200 nm).

Sprivivirus, Perhabdovirus, and *Vesciculovirus.* Rhabdovirus has been reported to cause acute disease in Rio Grande Perch (cichlid) and North American (Mexican) cichlid (*Cichlasoma cyanoguttatum*) [78]. These viruses are responsible for infections in a wide range of freshwater and marine fishes (*Anguilliformes, Clupeiformes, Cypriniformes, Gadiformes, Perciformes, Pleuronectiformes*, and *Salmoniformes*) [79].

Infections with three rhabdoviruses such as infectious hematopoietic necrosis (IHN), viral hemorrhagic septicemia (VHS), and spring viraemia of carp (SVC) are listed by OIE as notifiable diseases [31]. Fish rhabdoviruses generally show tissue

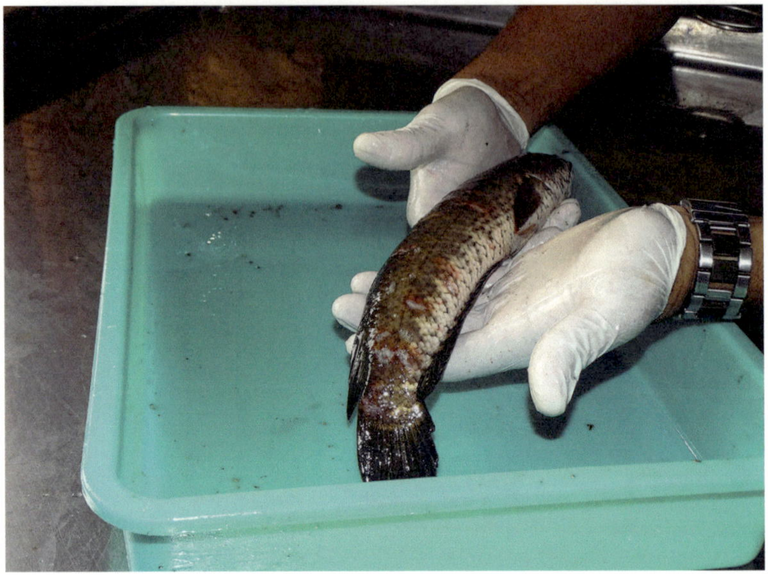

Figure 14.
Snakehead fish with surface ulcerations and hemorrhagic areas infected with snakehead rhabdovirus.

tropism to kidney, spleen, and brain while liver, heart, and gill are also found to be the multiplication sites albeit with low titers [80]. Rhabdoviruses were isolated from infected snakeheads (*Ophicephalus striatus*) from various Southeast Asian countries such as Thailand, Myanmar (Burma), and Philippines in 1980s and also from other epizootic ulcerative syndrome (EUS)-infected fishes [81–83]. Striped snakehead skin ulcerative disease reported in striped snakehead in Burma and Thailand caused large, deep ulcerations of the skin on the head and body of fish [82, 84]. Infected fish show signs of lethargy leading to mortality within 1 week [79]. Recently, isolation of a snakehead fish vesiculovirus (SHVV) was reported from hybrid catfish in China [85]. First report of emergence of a rhabdovirus (SHRV In) in India was from an infected snakehead that were undergoing mortality in the extensive type aquaculture tanks in the rural areas of South India that had behavioral abnormalities and surface ulcerations (**Figure 14**) [86]. Experimental infection with SHRV-In exhibited clinical signs of listlessness, uncoordinated spiral swimming, anorexia, lethargy, loss of scales, discoloration, small pale white patches on the body, hemorrhagic areas, and surface ulcers in juvenile snakeheads. Internally, fish showed hemorrhages and ascitic fluid [86].

4. Control measures

For successful aquaculture production, health management in the nursery, and grow-out culture is essential because the quality and quantity of fish produced depend on biosecurity and health management measures adopted by the aquaculturist. In general, fish are stocked at high densities in nurseries and grow-out farms and therefore, improper management can lead to weak fingerlings with low survival. Prevention is always considered as the first step in controlling infectious diseases in aqua farms. General biosecurity measures like sanitizing hands before handling fish, having foot dips with disinfectants at all entry points in the farm, disinfecting the source water are more important to prevent the frequent occurrence and spread of disease. Development of suitable preventive and control measures, specifically vaccines, immunostimulants, herbal extract, and probiotics are also of high significance, for the fish farmers to protect their crop against pathogens (**Tables 1–3**).

Disease	Pathogen	Vaccine type	Antigens/ targets	Delivery methods	Country/ region
Infectious spleen and kidney necrosis	ISKNV Iridovirus	Inactivated	Inactivated ISKNV	Intra peritoneal	Singapore
Redseabream iridovirus disease	RSIV iridovirus	Inactivated	Inactivated RSIV	Intraperitoneal	Japan
Viral nerves necrosis (VNN)	VNN Nodavirus	Recombinant	Recombinant VNN	Intraperitoneal	India
Koi ranaviral disease	KIRV Ranavirus	—	—	—	—
Similar damselfish viral disease	SRDV Ranavirus	—	—	—	—
Sleepy disease or carp edema virus disease	CEV Poxvirus	—	—	—	—
Tilapia lake virus	TiLV Tilapinevirus	—	—	—	—

Table 1.
Commercially available vaccines for viral diseases reported in India.

Viruses	Host	Immunostimulants
VHSV	Rainbow trout	*Marinobacter algicola* flagellins, ascorbic acid, ascorbate 2 monophosphate, Vit E
IHNV	Rainbow trout	Ascorbic acid and glucans
SVCV	Zebra fish	β glucans, LPS, polyinosinic: polycytidylic acid
IPNV	Atlantic salmon	Oligodeoxynucleotides (ODN) containing unmethylated CpG dinucleotides
GCHV	Grass carp	β glucans
KIRV	Common carp	Bacterial DNA (*A. hydrophila*)
EHNV	Cat fish	Methisoprinol
RSIV	Red sea bream	RsbIL-1β and RsbIL-8
ISKNV	Red drum	TO17
NNV	Grouper. Grouper, seven band grouper	Reishi immunomodulatory protein (riZ-8), Tryptophan & Whey and β-glucan

Table 2.
Experimental immunostimulants studied for fish viruses.

Virus	Species infected by the virus	Effective probiotic culture	Mode of action
IHNV	*O. mykiss*; *Oncorhynchus tshawytscha*; *O. nerka*	*Pseudomonas* sp.	Antiviral effect by blocking the sites of attachment for IHNV on the host. Proteolytic activity against various structural proteins of viruses affecting fish
LCDV	*Pleuronectes flews*; *Pleuronectes platessa*; *Acerina cernua*; *Cynoscion nothus*; *C. regalis*; *Bairdiella chrysura; Fundulus heteroclitus*	*Lactobacillus* sp. and *Lactobacillus sporogenes*, respectively	Perform as immunostimulants to boost innate immune response as well as disease resistance in opposition to LCDV
VHSV	*F. heteroclitus*; *Gasterosteus aculeatus*; *Salmo trutta*; *Morone saxatilis*; *Esox masquinongy*; *Oncorhynchus mykiss*; *Sprattus*; *Gadus morhua*	*Lactococcus lactis* (NZ3900)	*L. lactis* (NZ3900) constitutes G gene of VHSV under Nisin-controlled gene expression (NICE) system is utilized as an oral vaccine against the virus
KHV	*Cyprinus rubrofuscus*; *Cyprinus carpio*	Genetically engineered (GE) *Lactobacillus plantarum*	These are capable of expressing the ORF81 protein of KHV and act as oral vaccine
SVCV	*Cyprinus carpio*; *Ctenopharyngodon idella*; *Carassius auratus*; *Leuciscus idus*; *Tinca tinca*; *Notropis atherinoides*; *Hypophthalmichthys molitrix*	*L. plantarum*, *Bacillus velezensis*	It is capable of expressing the G protein of SVCV and can act as oral a vaccine to provide protection against SVCV
TiLV	*Oreochromis* spp	*Bacillus subtilis*, *Bacillus licheniformis*, and *B. pumilus*	Decreased viral load
OMV	*Oncorhynchus masou*; *Oncorhynchus nerka*; *Oncorhynchus keta*; *O. mykiss*; *Oncorhynchus kisutch*; etc.	*Pseudomonas* sp.	It produces a potent antiviral compound (46NW04A) that is effective against OMV

Table 3.
Probiotic bacteria used against viruses of fish.

5. Recent significant advances in research on the management of viral diseases

While there are successful vaccines available for many existing viral diseases, for emerging viral infections, development of vaccines is only in the preliminary stages [87, 88]. Since there is no commercial vaccine or effective antiviral treatment against SGIV infection currently, a high-throughput in vitro cell viability-based screening assay has been developed to find antiviral compounds against SGIV using the luminescent-based CellTiter-Glo reagent in cultured grouper spleen cells by quantificational measurement of the cytopathic effects induced by SGIV infection [89]. Aqueous preparations of the medicinal plant, *Viola philippica* has been found to have excellent inhibitory effects against Grouper iridovirus GIV during the viral infection stage of binding and replication in host cells [90]. Against SVCV, a total of 35 arctigenin derivatives have been synthesized and tested for their antiviral efficacy in EPC cells. Out of 35 derivatives screened, 32 were found to have a potential anti-SVCV effect at relatively high concentrations [91]. Additionally, a new coumarin derivative called 7-[6-(2-methylimidazole) hexyloxy] coumarin (D5) and imidazole coumarin derivative, 7-(4-benzimidazole-butoxy)-coumarin (BBC) have been synthesized and evaluated for the antiviral activity against spring viraemia of carp virus (SVCV), which showed that D5 and BBC had a strong antiviral activity SVCV expression in the host cells and in zebrafish [92–94]. Arctigenin (ARG) has also been found to have the highest inhibition on SVCV replication [95]. A novel coumarin derivative (C3007) could have significant potential for use as a therapeutic agent in aquatic systems and may also be appropriate for use in pond aquaculture environments to prevent viral transmission [96].

The arctigenin-imidazole hybrid derivative-15 with an eight-carbon atom linker length greatly suppressed apoptosis and the cellular morphological damage brought on by infectious hematopoietic necrosis virus (IHNV) in addition to decrease replication [97]. A new imidazole arctigenin derivative, 4-(8-(2-ethylimidazole) octyloxy)-arctigenin (EOA), significantly decreased cytopathic effect (CPE) and viral titer induced by IHNV in epithelioma papulosum correct as cyprini (EPC) cells. In addition, it significantly inhibited apoptosis induced by IHNV in EPC cells [98].

Since broad-spectrum water-immersion antiviral treatments are highly desirable, light-activated antivirals that target the viral membrane (envelope) of viruses have been developed to prevent viral-cell membrane fusion, ultimately blocking viral entry into cells [99]. An extract from *Ecklonia cava* has also been demonstrated for its ability to suppress VHSV in the fathead minnow (FHM) cell line and following oral administration to the olive flounder. Additionally, oral administration of the *E. cava* extract to the olive flounder increased the antiviral immune response and the efficacy of protection against VHSV, leading to the development of an antiviral status in the olive flounder [100]. Alpinone has been found to have in vitro antiviral activity against the infectious salmon anemia virus [101].

Drugs such as ammonium chloride and chlorpromazine hydrochloride drugs could be used for controlling nodavirus infection in aquaculture [102]. One of the best tools to prevent virus spread is the development of suitable vaccines. Binary ethylenimine (BEI) inactivated vaccine against the nervous necrosis virus has been generated and conferred partial protection to *Senegalese sole* when administered by intra-peritoneal injection, although they induced a different immune response [103]. An epitope-based vaccine (EBV) has also been developed using a computation approach for the first time and tested against seven banded grouper nervous necrosis virus [104].

Common disinfectants such as iodine, sodium hypochlorite, hydrogen peroxide, and formalin can be effectively used to reduce viral loads [105]. Therefore, the proper use of such disinfectants may be encouraged and put into practice in order to reduce the development of TiLV in aquaculture farms and related facilities. β-propiolactone inactivation of viral particles exhibited higher protection efficacy against virus challenge than formaldehyde [106]. When combined with the adjuvant Montanide IMS 1312 VG and booster immunizations, the β-propiolactone-inactivated vaccine provides a high level of protection from TiLV challenge in tilapia.

6. Conclusion

In India, aquaculture plays a key role in increasing production of highly nutritious and cheap protein to the masses while at the same time generating more employment opportunities. Emerging viral diseases of various categories are, however, causing great concern to the sector threatening the sustainability of aquaculture operations. A definite understanding of the etiological agents is therefore of paramount importance in generating interventions in controlling the diseases. Adequate diagnostic protocols and ability to detect different strains arising out of mutations resulting in emergent infections are also highly indispensable. Many of the viral disease agents detected in India showed variations from their global counter parts. It would be therefore essential to develop proper surveillance methods and systematic approach of documentation coupled with fast responsiveness to a reported infection to keep the emerging viral diseases under control. This would help in containing the infection and probably eliminating the incriminating agent if proper biosecurity principles are applied. Adequate care also needs to be given to the seed production of the candidate species by screening the brood stock so that the possible vertical transmission can be prevented. As the therapeutic measures are having little success with viral infections in fish, prophylactic measures, including vaccines, immunostimulants, herbal extracts and probiotics to protect the crop against viral diseases are to be extensively explored.

7. Future perspectives

Realizing the trend of increasing viral infections in fish, it is necessary to build adequate preventive measures to contain the spread of the disease. The requirements in this aspect include:

- A well-equipped diagnostic laboratory with appropriately trained and experienced staff to help in the diagnosis of virus-infected fish.

- Effective biosecurity measures by farmers to prevent infection from spreading to farmed fish.

- Comprehensive knowledge of the newly emerging and reemerging viral infections, current health management techniques, dynamics, infrastructure, and regulatory norms.

- Stocking fast-growing fish with the appropriate density and composition, integrating a system for effluent treatment and resource management and sanitizing the pond environment to increase aquaculture productivity.

- Modern health management practices developed on epidemiological principles with active and passive surveillance programme for advanced prediction of disease occurrence to protect the crop

- "National Surveillance Programme on Aquatic Animal Diseases (NSPAAD)" currently in vogue in India is already trying to address the issue of disease control in fish and shellfish species since 2013. It aims to record prevalence of diseases, incidence of emerging and remerging diseases and to develop immediate response measures to identify, notify and contain the diseases especially viral infections so that the situation is contained.

- Additionally, conducting fish health camps and awareness programme under the NSPAAD for the benefit of farmers to enable them to take precautionary measures before the disease spreads and become out of control.

Author details

Kollanoor Riji John[1*], Panchavarnam Sivasankar[2]
and Mulloorpeedikayil Rosalind George[1]

1 Kerala University of Fisheries and Ocean Studies, Kochi, India

2 Fisheries College and Research Institute, Thoothukudi, Tamil Nadu, India

*Address all correspondence to: rijijohn@gmail.com

References

[1] Raja K, Aanand P, Padmavathy S, Sampathkumar JS. Present and future market trends of Indian ornamental fish sector. Int. J. Fish. Aquat. Stud. 2019;**7**(2):6-15

[2] Bajpai V, Pragyan D, Suman K, Mohanty J, Sahoo PK. Viral diseases in Indian freshwater and marine water pisciculture. Current Science. 2022;**122**:261-280

[3] Sánchez-Paz A. White spot syndrome virus: An overview on an emergent concern. Veterinary Research. 2010;**41**(6):43. DOI: 10.1051/vetres/2010015

[4] Walker PJ, Winton JR. Emerging viral diseases of fish and shrimp. Veterinary Research. 2010;**41**(6):51. DOI: 10.1051/vetres/2010022

[5] Mohan CV, Bhatta R. Social and economic impacts of aquatic animal health problems on aquaculture in India. FAO Fisheries Technical Paper. 2002:63-75

[6] Bagum N, Monir MS, Khan MH. Present status of fish diseases and economic losses due to incidence of disease in rural freshwater aquaculture of Bangladesh. J Innov Dev Strategy. 2013;**7**:48-53

[7] Sahoo PK, Mohanty J, Garnayak JSK, Mohanty BR, Banya K. Estimation of loss due to argulosis in carp culture ponds in India. Indian Journal Fisheries. 2013;**60**:99-102

[8] Subasinghe RP, Bondad-Reantaso MG, McGladdery SE. Aquaculture development, health and wealth. In: Subasinghe RP, Reantaso MGB, McGladdery SE, editors. Aquaculture in the Third Millennium. Technical Proceedings of the Conference on Aquaculture in the Third Millennium, Bangkok. Bangkok, Thailand: Aquaculture in the Third Millennium; 2001. pp. 167-1914

[9] Bondad-Reantaso MG, Subasinghe RP, Arthur JR, Ogawa K, Chinabut S, Adlard R, Tan Z, Shariff M. Disease and health management in Asian aquaculture. Veterinary parasitology. 2005;30:249-272. DOI: 10.1016/j.vetpar.2005.07.005

[10] Karvonen A, Räihä V, Klemme I, Ashrafi R, Hyvärinen P, Sundberg LR. Quantity and quality of aquaculture enrichments influence disease epidemics and provide ecological alternatives to antibiotics. Antibiotics. 2021;**10**(3):335

[11] Sivasankar P, John KR, George MR, Mansoor MM, Kumar PM, Selvamagheswaran M, et al. Analysis of immune gene expression in seabass (*Lates calcarifer*) immunized with inactivated vaccine against similar damselfish virus. Indian Journal of Animal Research. 2021;**55**(1):31-39

[12] Mishra SS, Rakesh D, Dhiman M, Choudhary P, Debbarma J, Sahoo SN, et al. Present status of fish disease management in freshwater aquaculture in India: State-of-the-art-review. Journal of Aquaculture & Fisheries. 2017;**1**(3):14

[13] Mishra SS, Dhiman M, Swain P, Das BK. Fish diseases and health management issues in aquaculture. ICAR-CIFA Training manual. 2015;**18**:23-29

[14] George MR, John KR, Mansoor MM, Saravanakumar R, Sundar P, Pradeep V. Isolation and characterization of a ranavirus from koi, *Cyprinus carpio* L., experiencing mass mortalities in India. Journal of Fish

Diseases. 2015;38:389-403. DOI: 10.1111/jfd.12246

[15] Jancovich JK, Chinchar VG, Hyatt A, Miyazaki T, Williams T, Zhang QY. Family iridoviridae. In: King AMQ, Adams MJ, Carstens EB, Lefkowitz EJ, editors. Virus Taxonomy, Ninth Report of the International Committee on Taxonomy of Viruses. San Diego, CA: Elsevier; 2012. pp. 193-210

[16] Chinchar VG. Ranaviruses (family Iridoviridae): Emerging coldblooded killers. Archives of Virology. 2002;**147**:447-470

[17] Williams T, Barbosa-Solomieu V, Chinchar VG. A decade of advances in iridovirus research. Advances in Virus Research. 2005;**65**:173-248

[18] Ahne W, Bremont M, Hedrick RP, Hyatt AD, Whittington RJ. Iridoviruses associated with epizootic haematopoietic necrosis EHN in aquaculture. World Journal of Microbiology and Biotechnology. 1997;**13**:367-373

[19] Mao J, Hedrick RP, Chinchar VG. Molecular characterization, sequence analysis, and taxonomic position of newly isolated fish iridoviruses. Virology. 1997;**229**:212-220

[20] Qin QW, Chang SF, Ngoh-Lim GH, Gibson-Kueh S, Shi C, Lam TJ. Characterization of a novel ranavirus isolated from grouper *Epinephelus tauvina*. Diseases of Aquatic Organisms. 2003;**53**:1-9

[21] Zupanovic Z, Musso C, Lopez G, Louriero CL, Hyatt AD, Hengstberger S, et al. Isolation and characterization of iridoviruses from the giant toad Bufo marinus in Venezuela. Diseases of Aquatic Organisms. 1998;**33**:1-9

[22] Jancovich JK, Bremont M, Touchman JW, Jacobs BL. Evidence for multiple recent host species shifts among the Ranaviruses (family Iridoviridae). Journal of Virology. 2010;**84**:2636-2647

[23] Holopainen R, Ohlemeyer S, Sch€utze H, Bergmann SM, Tapiovaara H. Ranavirus phylogeny and differentiation based on major capsid protein, DNA polymerase and neurofilament triplet H1-like protein genes. Diseases of Aquatic Organisms. 2009;**85**:81-91

[24] Mao J, Wang J, Chinchar GD, Chinchar VG. Molecular characterization of a ranavirus isolated from largemouth bass Micropterus salmoides. Diseases of Aquatic Organisms. 1999;**37**:107-114

[25] Hyatt AD, Gould AR, Zupanovic Z, Cunningham AA, Hengstberger S, Whittington RJ, et al. Comparative studies of piscine and amphibian iridoviruses. Archives of Virology. 2000;**145**:301-331

[26] Whittington RJ, Becker JA, Dennis MM. Iridovirus infections in finfish—Critical review with emphasis on ranaviruses. Journal of Fish Diseases. 2010;**33**:95-122

[27] John KR, George MR, Kar D, Mansoor MM, Kumar PM, Singha R, et al. Detection of ranavirus infection in cultivated carps of Northeast India. Fish Pathology. 2016;**51**(Special-issue):S66-S74

[28] Sivasankar P, John KR, GeorgeMR, MageshkumarP, ManzoorMM, Jeyaseelan MP. Characterization of a virulent ranavirus isolated from marine ornamental fish in India. Virus Disease. 2017;**28**(4):373-382. DOI: 10.1007/s13337-017-0408-2

[29] Matsuoka S, Inouye K, Nakajima K. Cultured fish species affected by red sea bream iridoviral disease from 1991 to

1995. Fish Pathology. 1996;31(4):233-234. https://doi.org/10.3147/jsfp.31.233

[30] Kawakami H, Nakajima K. Cultured fish species affected by red sea bream iridoviral disease from 1996 to 2000. Fish Pathology. 2002;37(1):45-47. https://doi.org/10.3147/jsfp.37.45

[31] OIE 2019. On-line update of manual of diagnostic tests for aquatic animals. Available from: http://www.oieint/en/standard-setting/aquatic-manual/access-online/

[32] Girisha SK, Puneeth TG, Nithin MS, Kumar BN, Ajay SK, Vinay TN, et al. Red sea bream iridovirus disease (RSIVD) outbreak in Asian seabass (*Lates calcarifer*) cultured in open estuarine cages along the west coast of India: First report. Aquaculture. 2020;**520**:734712

[33] Nakajima K, Maeno Y. Pathogenicity of red sea bream iridovirus and other fish iridoviruses to red sea bream. Fish Pathol. 1998;**33**:143-144

[34] Puneeth TG, Baliga P, Girisha SK, Shekar M, Nithin MS, Suresh T, et al. Complete genome analysis of a red seabream iridovirus (RSIV) isolated from Asian seabass (Lates *calcarifer*) in India. Virus Research. 2021;**291**:198199

[35] Guo CJ, Wu YY, Yang LS, Yang XB, He J, Mi S, et al. Infectious spleen and kidney necrosis virus (a fish iridovirus) enters Mandarin fish fry cells via caveola-dependent endocytosis. Journal of virology. 2012;**86**(5):2621-2631. DOI: 10.1128/JVI.06947-11

[36] He JG, Weng SP, Huang ZJ, Zeng K. Identification of outbreak and infectious diseases pathogen of *Siniperca chuatsi*. Acta Sceintiarum Naturalium Universitatis Sunyatseni. 1998;**37**:74-77

[37] He JG, Zeng K, Weng SP, Chan SM. Experimental transmission, pathogenicity and physical–chemical properties of infectious spleen and kidney necrosis virus (ISKNV). Aquaculture 2002;204:11-24. DOI: 10.1016/S0044-8486(01)00639-1

[38] Girisha SK, Kushala KB, Nithin MS, Puneeth TG, Naveen Kumar BT, Vinay TN, et al. First report of the infectious spleen and kidney necrosis virus (ISKNV) infection in ornamental fishes in India. Transboundary and emerging diseases. 2021;**68**(2):964-972

[39] Jung-Schroers V, Adamek M, Wohlsein P, Wolter J, Wedekind H, Steinhagen D. First outbreak of an infection with infectious spleen and kidney necrosis virus (ISKNV) in ornamental fish in Germany. Diseases of Aquatic Organisms. 2016;**119**(3):239-244. DOI: 10.3354/dao02995

[40] Yanong RPE, Waltzek TB. Megalocytivirus Infections in Fish, With Emphasis on Ornamental Species 1. What Are the Megalocytiviruses? University of Florida: University of Florida IFAS Extension; 2012

[41] Jeong JB, Kim HY, Jun LJ, Lyu JH, Park NG, Kim JK, et al. Outbreaks and risks of infectious spleen and kidney necrosis virus disease in freshwater ornamental fishes. Diseases of Aquatic Organisms. 2008;**78**(3):209-215. DOI: 10.3354/dao01879

[42] Shahi N, Mallik SK, Kala K, Joshi N, Patiyal RS, Chandra S, et al. Seasonal emergence of benign epidermal tumor in farm-reared adult grass carp (*Ctenopharyngodon idella*) caused by lymphocystis disease virus at Uttarakhand, India. Aquaculture. 2020;**526**:735408. DOI: 10.1016/j.aquaculture.2020.735408

[43] Hartman KH, Yanong RPE, Pouder DB, Petty BD, Francis-Floyd R, Riggs AC, et al. Koi Herpesvirus Disease (KHVD). Gainesville, Florida: IFAS Extension, University of Florida; 2013. pp. 1-9. DOI: org/10.32473/edis-vm113-2013

[44] Murakami Y, Shitanaka M, Toshida S, Matsuzato T. Studies on mass mortality of juvenile carp: About mass mortality showing edema. Bull Hiroshima Fresh Water Fish Exp Stn. 1976;**32**(2):19-33

[45] Swaminathan TR, Kumar R, Dharmaratnam A, Basheer VS, Sood N, Pradhan PK, et al. Emergence of carp edema virus in cultured ornamental koi carp, *Cyprinus carpio* koi, in India. Journal of General Virology. 2016;**97**(12):3392-3399. DOI: 10.1099/jgv.0.000649

[46] Sahoo PK, Pattanayak S, Paul A, Sahoo MK, Kumar P. Carp edema virus in ornamental fish farming in India: A potential threat to koi carps but not to co-cultured Indian major carp or goldfish. Indian Journal of Experimental Biology. 2020;**58**:254-262

[47] Oyamatsu T, Matoyama H, Yamamoto K, Fukuda H. A trial for detection of carp edema virus by using polymerase chain reaction. Aquaculture Science. 1997;45(2):247-251. https://doi.org/10.11233/aquaculturesci1953.45.247

[48] Miyazaki T, Isshiki T, Katsuyuki H. Histopathological and electron microscopy studies on sleepy disease of koi *Cyprinus carpio koi* in Japan. Diseases of aquatic organisms. 2005;**65**(3):197-207. DOI: 10.3354/dao065197

[49] Hesami S, Viadanna P, Steckler N, Spears S, Thompson P, Kelley K, Waltzek T. Carp Edema Virus Disease (CEVD)/Koi Sleepy Disease (KSD). University of Florida EDIS Publication FA189:1-6 [Internet]. 2015: Available from: https://edis.ifas.ufl.edu/pdffiles/FA/FA18900.pdf. [Accessed January 21, 2022]

[50] Bandin I, Souto S. Betanodavirus and VER disease: A 30-year research review. Pathogens. 2020;**9**:106. DOI: 10.3390/pathogens9020106

[51] Breuil G, Bonami JR, Pepin JF, Pichot Y. Viral infection (picorna-like virus) associated with mass mortalities in hatchery-reared sea-bass (*Dicentrarchus labrax*) larvae and juveniles. Aquaculture 1991;15:109-116. DOI: 10.1016/0044-8486(91)90258-9

[52] Glazebrook JS, Heasman MP, De Beer SW. Picorna-like viral particles associated with mass mortalities in larval barramundi, *Lates calcarifer* Bloch. Journal of Fish Diseases. 1990;**13**:245-249. DOI: 10.1111/j.1365-2761.1990.tb00780.x

[53] Mori KI, Nakai T, Muroga K, Arimoto M, Mushiake K, Furusawa I. Properties of a new virus belonging to *Nodaviridae* found in larval striped jack (*Pseudocaranx dentex*) with nervous necrosis. Virology 1992;187(1):368-371. https://doi.org/10.1016/0042-6822(92)90329-N

[54] Nopadon P, Aranya P, Tipaporn T, Toshihiro N, Takayuki K, Masashi M, et al. Nodavirus associated with pathological changes in adult spotted coral groupers (*Plectropomus maculatus*) in Thailand with viral nervous necrosis. Research in veterinary science. 2009;**87**(1):97-101. DOI: 10.1016/j.rvsc.2009.01.004

[55] Frerichs GN, Rodger HD, Peric Z. Cell culture isolation of piscine neuropathy nodavirus from juvenile sea bass, *Dicentrarchus labrax*. J. Gen. Virol. 1996;**77**:2067-2071

[56] Leong J. Fish viruses. In: Mahy BWJ, Van Regenmortel MHV, editors.

Encyclopedia of Virology. Third ed, 5 Vols. Oxford: Elsevier; 2008. pp. 227-234

[57] World Organization for Animal Health (OIE). Manual of diagnostic tests for aquatic animals. Chapter 2.3.12. Viral Encephalopathy and Retinopathy. 2019. pp. 1-20. Available from: https://www.woah.org/fileadmin/Home/eng/Health_standards/aahm/current/chapitre_viral_encephalopathy_retinopathy.pdf

[58] Jithendran KP, Shekhar MS, Kannappan S, Azad IS. Nodavirus infection in freshwater ornamental fishes in India: Diagnostic histopathology and nested RT-PCR. Asian Fisheries Science. 2011;**24**:12-19

[59] Hata N, Okinaka Y, Iwamoto T, Kawato Y, Mori KI, Nakai T. Identification of RNA regions that determine temperature sensitivities in betanodaviruses. Archives of Virology. 2010;**155**(10):1597-1606

[60] Nguyen HD, Nakai T, Muroga K. Progression of striped jack nervous necrosis virus (SJNNV) infection in naturally and experimentally infected striped jack *Pseudocaranx dentex* larvae. Diseases of Aquatic Organisms. 1996;**24**(2):99-105

[61] Le Breton A, Grisez L, Sweetman J, Ollevier F. Viral nervous necrosis (VNN) associated with mass mortalities in cage-reared sea bass, *Dicentrarchus labrax* (L.). Journal of Fish Diseases. 1997;**20**(2):145-151

[62] Gomez DK, Lim DJ, Baeck GW, Youn HJ, Shin NS, Youn HY, et al. Detection of betanodaviruses in apparently healthy aquarium fishes and invertebrates. Journal of Veterinary Science. 2006;7(4):369-374. DOI: 10.4142/jvs.2006.7.4.369

[63] Nazari A, Hassan MD, Bovo G, Zorriehzahra MJ, Azmi TI, Arshad SS. Pathogenicity of viral nervous necrosis virus for Guppy fish, *Poecilia reticulata*. Iranian Journal of Fisheries Sciences. 2014;**13**(1):168-177

[64] John KR, George MR, Jeyatha B, Saravanakumar R, Sundar P, Jithendran KP, Koppang EO. Isolation and characterization of Indian betanodavirus strain from infected farm-reared Asian seabass *Lates calcarifer* (Bloch, 1790) juveniles. Aquaculture research. 2014;45:1481-1488. DOI: 10.1111/are.12095

[65] Eyngor M, Zamostiano R, Kembou Tsofack JE, Berkowitz A, Bercovier H, Tinman S, Lev M, Hurvitz A, Galeotti M, Bacharach E, Eldar A. Identification of a novel RNA virus lethal to tilapia. Journal of clinical microbiology. 2014;52: 4137-4146. DOI: 10.1128/JCM.00827-14

[66] Aich N, Paul A, Choudhury, TG, Saha H. Tilapia lake virus (TiLV) disease: Current status of understanding. Aquaculture and Fisheries. 2022;7: 7-17. DOI: 10.1016/j.aaf.2021.04.007

[67] Bacharach E, Mishra N, Briese T, Zody MC, Kembou Tsofack JE, Zamostiano R, et al. Characterization of a novel orthomyxo-like virus causing mass die-offs of tilapia. MBio. 2016;7:e00431-16 10.1128/mBio.00431-16

[68] Adams MJ, Lefkowitz EJ, King AM, Harrach B, Harrison RL, Knowles NJ, et al. Changes to taxonomy and the International Code of Virus Classification and Nomenclature ratified by the International Committee on Taxonomy of Viruses. Archives of virology. 2017;**162**(8):2505-2538

[69] Behera BK, Pradhan PK, Swaminathan TR, Sood N, Paria P, Das A, et al. Emergence of tilapia lake virus associated with mortalities of farmed Nile tilapia *Oreochromis niloticus* (Linnaeus 1758) in India. Aquaculture. 2018;**484**:168-174

[70] Jaemwimol P, Rawiwan P, Tattiyapong P, Saengnual P, Kamlangdee A, Surachetpong W. Susceptibility of important warm water fish species to tilapia lake virus (TiLV) infection. Aquaculture 2018;497:462-468. DOI: 10.1016/j.aquaculture.2018.08.028

[71] Surachetpong W, Janetanakit T, Nonthabenjawan N, Tattiyapong P, Sirikanchana K, Amonsin A. Outbreaks of tilapia lake virus infection, Thailand, 2015-2016. Emerging Infectious Diseases. 2017;**23**:1031-1033. DOI: 10.3201/eid2306.161278

[72] Tsofack JEK, Zamostiano R, Watted S, Berkowitz A, Rosenbluth E, Mishra N, et al. Detection of tilapia lake virus in clinical samples by culturing and nested reverse transcription-PCR. Journal of Clinical Microbiology. 2017;**55**:759-767. DOI: 10.1128/JCM.01808-16

[73] Dong HT, Ataguba GA, Khunrae P, Rattanarojpong T, Senapin S. Evidence of TiLV infection in tilapia hatcheries from 2012 to 2017 reveals probable global spread of the disease. Aquaculture. 2017;**479**:579-583. DOI: 10.1016/j.aquaculture.2017.06.035

[74] Mugimba KK, Lamkhannat M, Dubey S, Mutoloki S, Munang'andu HM, Evensen Ø. Tilapia lake virus downplays innate immune responses during early stage of infection in Nile tilapia (*Oreochromis niloticus*). Scientific Reports 2020;10(1):1-2. https://doi.org/10.1038/s41598-020-73781-y

[75] Swaminathan TR, Nithyanantham SR, Narendrakumar L, Dharmaratnam A, Sood N, Pradhan PK, et al. Co-infection of *Lactococcus garvieae* and Tilapia lake virus (TiLV) in Nile tilapia *Oreochromis niloticus* cultured in India. Diseases of Aquatic Organisms. 2021;**147**:127-140. DOI: 10.3354/dao03638

[76] Walker PJ, Blasdell KR, Calisher CH, Dietzgen RG, Kondo H, Kurath G, et al. ICTV virus taxonomy profile: Rhabdoviridae. Journal of General Virology. 2018;**99**(4):447-448

[77] Dale JL, Peters D. Protein composition of the virions of five rhabdovirus. Intervirology. 1981;**16**:86-94

[78] Essbauer S, Ahne W. Viruses of lower vertebrates. Journal of Veterinary Medicine, Series B. 2001;48:403-475. DOI: 10.1046/j.1439-0450.2001.00473.x

[79] Malsberger RG, Lautenslager G. Fish viruses: Rhabdovirus isolated from a species of the family Cichlidae [Rio Grande perch (*Cichlasoma cyanoguttatum*)]. Fish Health News. 1980

[80] Lovy J, Lewis NL, Hershberger PK, Bennett W, Meyers TR, Garver KA. Viral tropism and pathology associated with viral hemorrhagic septicemia in larval and juvenile Pacific herring. Veterinary Microbiology. 2012;**161**(1-2):66-76

[81] Frerichs GN, Millar SD, Roberts RJ. Ulcerative rhabdovirus in fish in South-East Asia. Nature. 1986;**322**(6076):216. DOI: 10.1038/322216a0

[82] Ahne W, Jørgensen PV, Olesen NJ, Wattanavijarn W. Serological examination of a rhabdovirus isolated from snakehead (*Ophicephalus striatus*) in Thailand with ulcerative syndrome. Journal of Applied Ichthyology. 1988;4:194-196. DOI: 10.1111/j.1439-0426.1988.tb00562.x

[83] John KR, George MR. Viruses associated with epizootic ulcerative syndrome, an update. Ind. J. Virol. 2012;**23**:106-113

[84] Frerichs GN, Hill BJ, Way K. Ulcerative disease rhabdovirus: Cell-line susceptibility and serological

comparison with other fish rhabdoviruses. Journal of Fish Diseases. 1989;12:51-56. DOI: 10.1111/j.1365-2761.1989.tb01290.x

[85] Zeng W, Wang Q, Wang Y, Liu C, Liang H, Fang X, et al. Genomic characterization and taxonomic position of a rhabdovirus from a hybrid snakehead. Archives of virology. 2014;**159**(9):2469-2473

[86] John KR, George MR, Mageshkumar P, Mansoor MM, Kaviarasu D, Sivasankar P, et al. Isolation and characterisation of a novel rhabdovirus from snakehead fish showing surface ulcerations and mortality from India: First report. Aquaculture. 2021;**544**:737120. DOI: 10.1016/j.aquaculture.2021.737120

[87] Dhar AK, Manna SK, Allnutt FT. Viral vaccines for farmed finfish. Virus Dis. 2014;**25**:1-7. DOI: 10.1007/s13337-013-0186-4

[88] Ma J, Bruce TJ, Jones EM, Cain KD. A review of fish vaccine development strategies: Conventional methods and modern biotechnological approaches. Microorganisms. 2019;7(11):569. DOI: 10.3390/microorganisms7110569

[89] Jia K, Yuan Y, Liu W, Liu L, Qin Q, Yi M. Identification of inhibitory compounds against Singapore grouper iridovirus infection by cell viability-based screening assay and droplet digital PCR. Marine Biotechnology. 2018;**20**:35-44

[90] Yu Q, Liu M, Xiao H, Wu S, Qin X, Lu Z, et al. The inhibitory activities and antiviral mechanism of *Viola philippica* aqueous extracts against grouper iridovirus infection in vitro and in vivo. Journal of Fish Diseases. 2019;**42**:859-868

[91] Chen WC, Hu Y, Liu L, Shen YF, Wang GX, Zhu B. Synthesis and in vitro activities evaluation of arctigenin derivatives against spring viraemia of carp virus. Fish & Shellfish Immunology. 2018;**82**:17-26

[92] Chen WC, Liu L, Shen YF, Hu Y, Ling F, Wang GX, et al. A new coumarin derivative plays a role in rhabdoviral clearance by interfering glycoprotein function during the early stage of viral infection. Cellular Signalling. 2018;**51**:199-210

[93] Shen YF, Liu L, Feng CZ, Hu Y, Chen C, Wang GX, et al. Synthesis and antiviral activity of a new coumarin derivative against spring viraemia of carp virus. Fish & Shellfish Immunology. 2018;**81**:57-66

[94] Liu L, Hu Y, Lu J, Wang G. An imidazole coumarin derivative enhances the antiviral response to spring viremia of carp virus infection in zebrafish. Virus Research. 2019;**263**:112-118

[95] Shen YF, Liu L, Chen WC, Hu Y, Zhu B, Wang GX. Evaluation on the antiviral activity of arctigenin against spring viraemia of carp virus. Aquaculture. 2018;**483**:252-262

[96] Liu L, Qiu TX, Song DW, Shan LP, Chen J. Inhibition of a novel coumarin on an aquatic rhabdovirus by targeting the early stage of viral infection demonstrates potential application in aquaculture. Antiviral Research. 2020;**174**:104672

[97] Hu Y, Liu L, Li B, Shen Y, Wang GX, Zhu B. Synthesis of arctigenin derivatives against infectious hematopoietic necrosis virus. European Journal of Medicinal Chemistry. 2019;**163**:183-194

[98] Hu Y, Chen WC, Shen YF, Zhu B, Wang GX. Synthesis and antiviral activity of a new arctigenin derivative against IHNV in vitro and in vivo. Fish & Shellfish Immunology. 2019;**92**:736-745

[99] Balmer BF, Getchell RG, Powers RL, Lee J, Zhang T, Jung ME, et al. Broad-spectrum antiviral JL122 blocks infection and inhibits transmission of aquatic rhabdoviruses. Virology. 2018;**525**:143-149

[100] Yang HK, Jung MH, Avunje S, Nikapitiya C, Kang SY, Ryu YB, et al. Efficacy of algal Ecklonia cava extract against viral hemorrhagic septicemia virus (VHSV). Fish & Shellfish Immunology. 2018;**72**:273-281

[101] Valenzuela B, Rodrıguez FE, Modak B, Imarai M. Alpinone exhibited immunomodulatory and antiviral activities in Atlantic salmon. Fish & Shellfish Immunology. 2018;**74**:76-83

[102] Sushila N, Hameed ASS, Prasad KP, Majeed SA, Tripathi G. In vitro screening of selected antiviral drugs against betanodavirus. Journal of Virological Methods. 2018;**259**:66-73

[103] Valero Y, Olveira JG, Vázquez CL, Dopazo CP, Bandin I. BEI inactivated vaccine induces innate and adaptive responses and elicits partial protection upon reassortant betanodavirus infection in Senegalese sole. Vaccine. 2021;**9**(5):458

[104] Joshi A, Pathak DC, Mannan MA, Kaushik V. In-silico designing of epitope-based vaccine against the seven banded grouper nervous necrosis virus affecting fish species. Netw Model Anal Health Inform Bioinform. 2021. DOI: 10:37. https://doi.org/10.1007/s13721-021-00315-5

[105] Jaemwimol P, Sirikanchana K, Tattiyapong P, Mongkolsuk S, Surachetpong W. Virucidal effects of common disinfectants against tilapia lake virus. Journal of Fish Diseases. 2019;**42**(10):1383-1389

[106] Zeng W, Wang Y, Hu H, Wang Q, Bergmann SM, Wang Y, et al. Cell culture-derived tilapia lake virus-inactivated vaccine containing montanide adjuvant provides high protection against viral challenge for tilapia. Vaccine. 2021;**9**:86